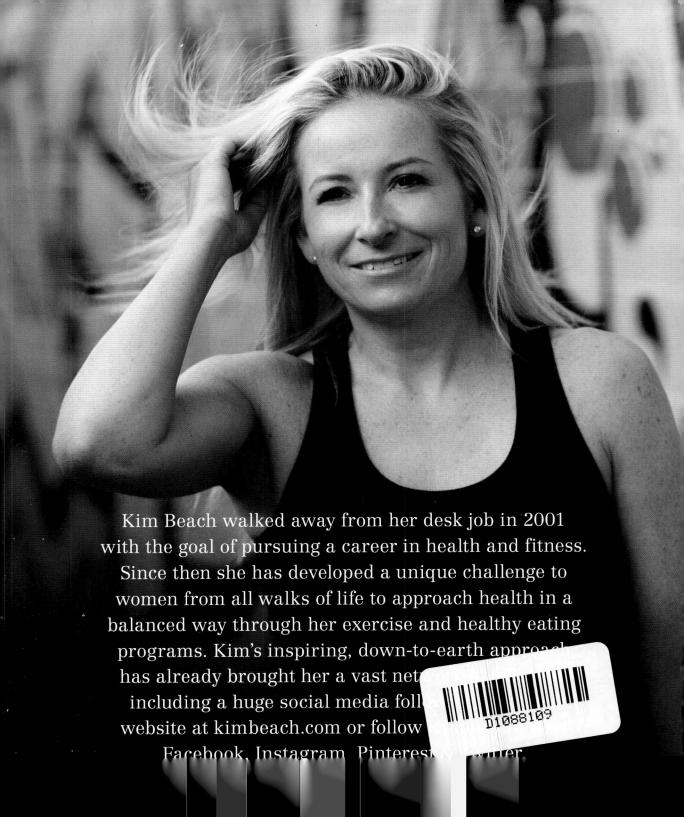

Kim Beach walked away from her desk job in 2001 with the goal of pursuing a career in health and fitness. Since then she has developed a unique challenge to women from all walks of life to approach health in a balanced way through her exercise and healthy eating programs. Kim's inspiring, down-to-earth approach has already brought her a vast net[work] including a huge social media foll[owing] website at kimbeach.com or follow [her] Facebook, Instagram, Pinterest [and Twitter.]

D1088109

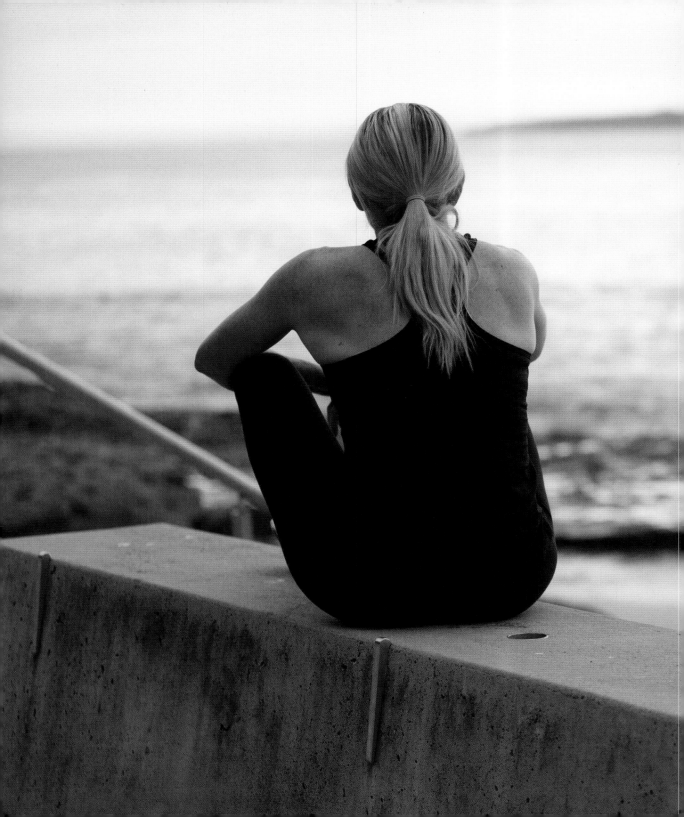

Kim Beach *x*

BEACH *FIT*

ABC
Books

NOTE

The content is not intended as a substitute for professional medical advice, diagnosis or treatment. If you have any specific questions about any medical matter, you should consult your doctor or other professional healthcare provider.

 The ABC 'Wave' device is a trademark of the Australian Broadcasting Corporation and is used under licence by HarperCollins*Publishers* Australia.

First published in Australia in 2017
by HarperCollins*Publishers* Australia Pty Limited
ABN 36 009 913 517
harpercollins.com.au

HarperCollins*Publishers*
Level 13, 201 Elizabeth Street, Sydney NSW 2000, Australia
Unit D1, 63 Apollo Drive, Rosedale, Auckland 0632, New Zealand
A 53, Sector 57, Noida, UP, India
1 London Bridge Street, London, SE1 9GF, United Kingdom
2 Bloor Street East, 20th floor, Toronto, Ontario M4W 1A8, Canada
195 Broadway, New York NY 10007, USA

National Library of Australia Cataloguing-in-Publication data:

Beach, Kim, author.
Beach fit: from the health and fitness expert who has helped thousands / Kim Beach.
978 0 7333 3787 1 (paperback)
Physical fitness–Popular works.
Health–Popular works.
Weight loss–Popular works.
Diet–Popular works.

Cover design by Lisa White, HarperCollins Design Studio and Jane Waterhouse
Internal design by Jane Waterhouse
Photography by Steve Baccon
Recipe photos by John Beach
Background textures by shutterstock.com
Colour reproduction by Graphic Print Group, South Australia
Printed and bound in China by RR Donnelley

The papers used by HarperCollins in the manufacture of this book are a natural, recyclable product made from wood grown in sustainable plantation forests. The fibre source and manufacturing processes meet recognised international environmental standards, and carry certification.

6 5 4 3 2   17 18 19 20

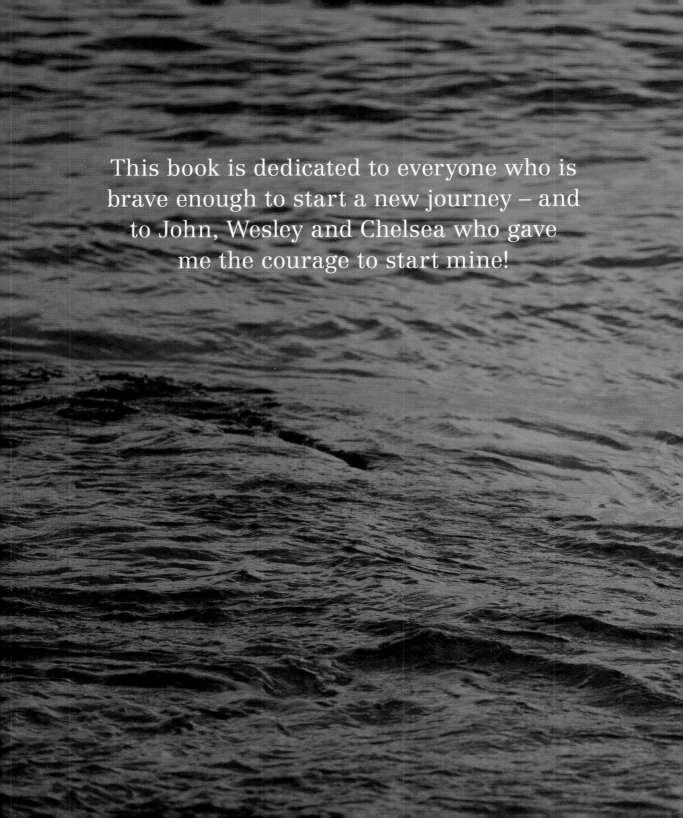

This book is dedicated to everyone who is brave enough to start a new journey – and to John, Wesley and Chelsea who gave me the courage to start mine!

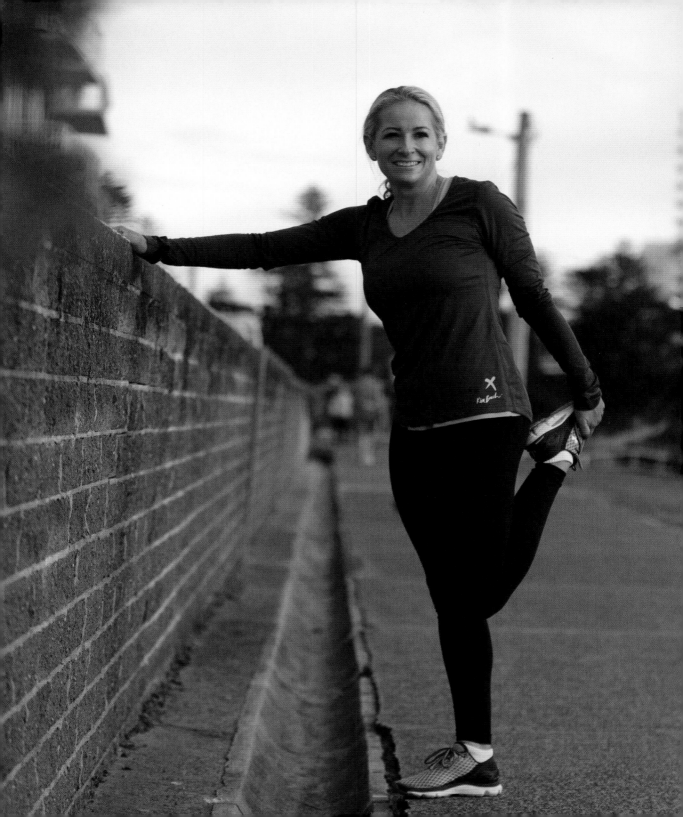

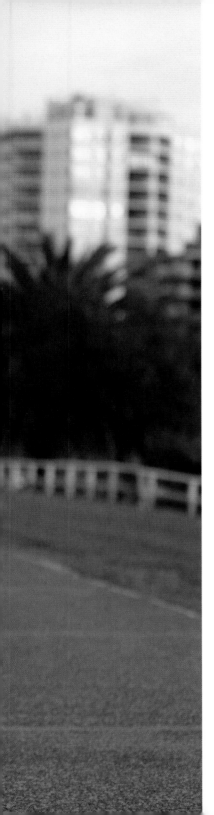

CONTENTS

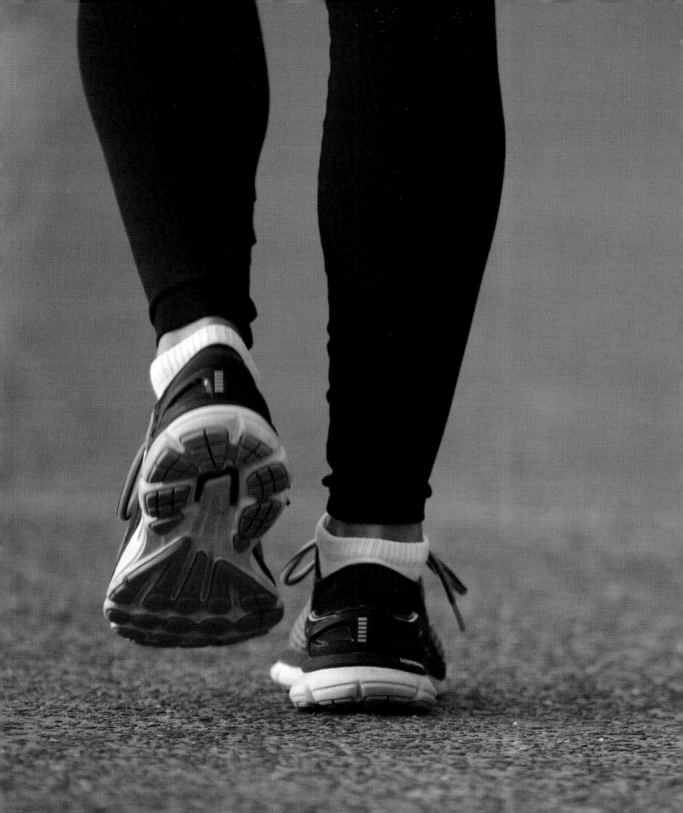

FOREWORD

I'm a doctor of patient safety, and I work full time as a director in a national health and human services practice. Well, I say full time, but sometimes it's actually more than full time, as in reality there are days when I'm up at 4am, on a plane at 6am, and home at 8pm. When I'm not travelling, I spend my days reviewing hospitals and health services. I absolutely love my job, but it can take its toll on the time I can spend exercising and planning my meals.

I've never really struggled with my weight, but life, and a few events, piled up and I ended up weighing more than I had when I was nine months' pregnant. Not only was I juggling a busy job as a health professional, but our kids moved out and it was just so easy to grab a takeaway for dinner. I thought I could compensate by picking up my exercise, but then I tore my hamstring (not exercising: doing a cartwheel on the beach!). Exercise was all a bit too hard, and when Christmas came along, I realised that I had literally nothing to wear for our Christmas lunch. I had slowly and steadily put on 12 kilos and gone up two dress sizes, from a 10 to a 14. I felt flat and really disappointed in myself, and with the big 50 a few short years away, I knew I had to do something to take back control and focus on my health.

I looked at a few programs; I really wanted something that was practical, sustainable, based on sound nutrition and easy to follow. I also needed something flexible that would fit in with my lifestyle and work commitments. As it was a few days after Christmas, and I had made a decision to start a program, I didn't want to wait for a scheduled program in the New Year (in case I lost my motivation!). I also knew that with my work I didn't have a set few nights a week to attend training, classes or meetings. I saw Kim's program on Facebook and downloaded a sample day on the program. It seemed to fit everything I was looking for, plus the #noexcuses name fit me to a tee, as all I had been doing was making excuses. This was no fad, Hollywood-style, eat-nothing, drink-shakes type of diet, and the exercise program looked completely manageable, flexible, and easy to do in the gym or at home. I signed up, went shopping and started the next day.

I followed Kim's eight-week program to the nth degree. At first I thought I was eating too much food, as there are a number of small meals throughout the day, but after Week One I could already see the results. The meals are really simple to prepare, and I was able to get most of the week's meals ready on a Sunday afternoon. The use of a sandwich press to cook pretty much everything was a revelation to me, and cut down cooking time dramatically. Simple things like drinking litres of water a day, replacing rice at dinner with cauliflower rice, having zucchini noodles instead of pasta, and eggwhite-only omelettes, meant that I was never hungry and always eating nutritious food. Having the exercise program set out each day made it so easy to follow, especially with the pictures for guidance!

I was so happy with my results. At the end of eight weeks I went from struggling to jog for five minutes to running five kilometres, I managed to climb the stairs at work without being breathless, I could do push-ups and squats and, despite having never been into the weight room at the gym, I'd mastered all the weight stations. The exercise was so much easier without the extra kilos; I was sleeping better, had so much more energy– even my skin looked amazing. I lost 10.6 kilos in eight weeks and my size 10 clothes are loose. My husband also lost 10 kilos, as I replaced his burger and chips for lunch with a big salad every day and we both had a meal from the program every night.

After finishing the program, I have lost an additional 1.5 kilos, and have managed to keep it off for the four months since I finished. The principles of the program are simple to follow and easy to sustain. Kim's 80:20 principle is my new mantra: I understand the types of food to eat and when to eat, and, even when eating out, I can always find something to suit. I now hate missing an exercise session, instead of hating to do one.

I was fortunate enough to meet Kim recently and tell her how she has transformed my approach to nutrition and exercise. Her positive outlook and encouragement have been invaluable to me. She's taught me that it's okay to have a bad day (or a few bad days), and brush yourself off and keep going without derailing your whole program: this is a lifestyle change and not a fad diet, and balance is the key.

I would encourage anyone wanting to lose weight, improve their fitness or just live a healthier life to have a look at Kim's programs. I know what it's like to be busy, but none of us should be too busy to focus on our health and fitness. Kim's approach is simple, sustainable and, believe me, you can follow it, no matter how busy you are!

Dr Bernadette Eather (RN, GCICU, MHM, DN)

'Be consistent, be brave, be tough, be disciplined, be focused, be passionate, be determined, be intense, be organised, be yourself, be amazing.'

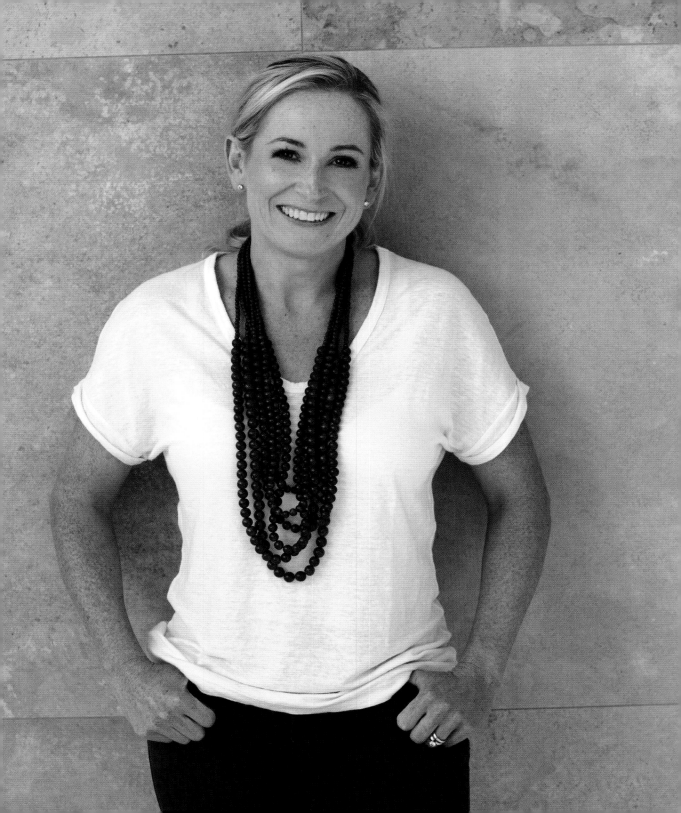

INTRODUCTION

HOW I GOT INTO HEALTH AND FITNESS ... EVENTUALLY!

If there is one lesson I have learned the hard way over the years, it's that you have to trust your own instincts and truly believe in yourself if you want to bring your dreams to life.

I clearly remember a conversation with my Year 10 careers advisor that had a massive impact on my life. At the time, it set me on a career path I wasn't comfortable with and, if I hadn't turned this around and followed my heart and my true passion for health and fitness, things could have turned out very differently for me!

The year was 1993. Let's call the teacher 'Mr Smith'.

> *Mr Smith*: 'So, Kim, what do you want to do with your life?'
> *Kim*: 'I want to be involved in something to do with health, fitness or sport.'
> *Mr Smith*: 'I am sorry Kim, but you simply do not have the marks for that.'
> *Kim*: 'Wow,' (feeling a little deflated at this point), 'okay ... what would you suggest then?'
> *Mr Smith*: 'Looking at your results and your excellent typing skills I suggest an office receptionist role would be a fantastic job for you.'

I remember walking away from the meeting with Mr Smith feeling upset. At the age of 15, I guess I didn't know any better, so I resigned myself to a career in administration. There is, of course, nothing wrong with a career in administration, but looking back I should have known it wasn't for me.

I was on every sports team in high school and was training for swimming twice a day, but as far as a career was concerned I was starting to get used to the idea that an office job was the next step for me. I did two more years of high school and then, with Mr Smith's suggested career path in front of me, I enrolled in a one-year, full-time office administration course. I passed the course with flying colours and was soon into my first job in Mascot, Sydney.

I was 19 and I had just landed my first full-time job and had taken the big step of buying my first car. On the outside my life looked perfect, but on the inside it was killing me.

Six months into my second job, as a typist for a major bank, I finally had THAT moment! I was angry, frustrated and unhappy, and I made a decision right then and there that I was going to leave and find a fresh start in the world of health and fitness.

I know that Mr Smith was just doing his job but it had finally dawned on me that what other people say or tell you to do is not important. You have to follow your own dreams and passions and do what makes you happy. For me, this meant going back to school at the age of 21. I enrolled in a two-year, full-time Diploma in Fitness at my local TAFE and I was determined to become a personal trainer!

Looking back now, I feel so lucky to have had such a supportive and loving family around me, who stood by my decision to walk away from a stable and growing career in office administration so I could become a personal trainer. From the moment I walked into Loftus TAFE on day one, I knew I had made the decision that I should have made years ago.

I loved every second of it and I couldn't get enough of learning about health, fitness and how the human body works. I never missed a minute of my classes, absorbing everything I could and learning from some amazing educators, some of whom I still consider my friends today.

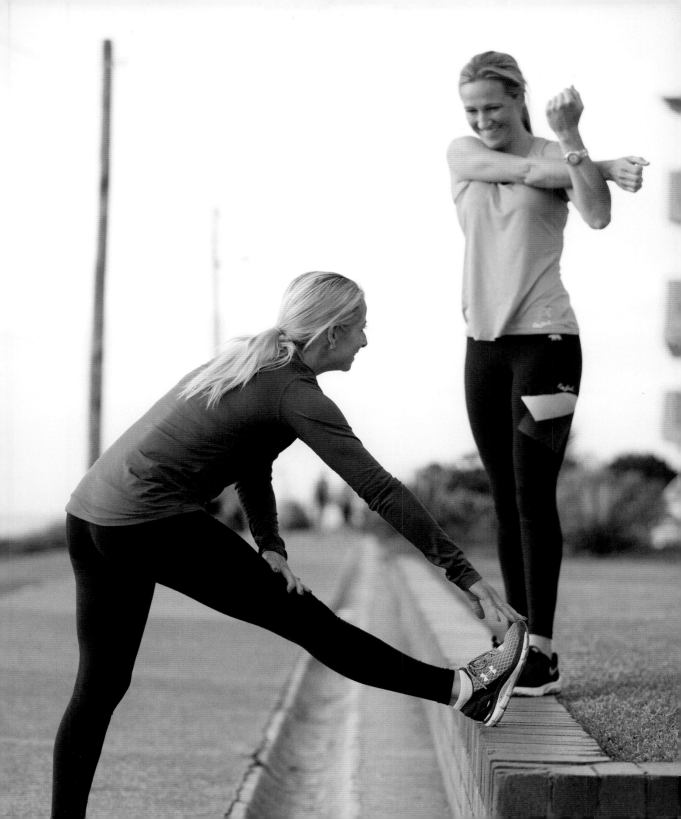

This period of study also ignited my passion for reading and today you will still find four to five books beside my bed, as I continue my learning about health, fitness and nutrition. I often laugh to myself when I am on holiday somewhere sitting around the pool and I am the only person excitedly reading the latest book on nutrition!

I am very proud to say I finished my Diploma in Fitness, receiving an award for best student in our class. I was 23 years old and finally ready to take on the world doing something that I really loved!

One of my TAFE lecturers set up an interview for me with Andrew Simmons and Geoff Jowett, the owners of Vision Personal Training, who had just opened their first studio in Caringbah, NSW. I have to admit to feeling a little nervous at the interview, sitting across from these two experienced trainers, and I thought I had definitely blown it when they asked me who my role model was and I blurted out 'Kylie Minogue'! I do love Kylie but it probably wasn't the right answer given the circumstances.

I must have said something right, however, because I got the job and was finally starting the career of my dreams. The hours were intense but the satisfaction I got on a daily basis from helping people lose weight and improve their health and fitness was truly exhilarating.

It was amazing to finally put everything I had learnt in my studies into practice. I had a lot of different clients, all with different goals. Some wanted to lose weight, others wanted to become leaner, fitter, healthier or stronger. Every day I was learning in practical terms and even though my work was focused on training people physically, I started to realise that correct nutrition was actually the key to people achieving their health and fitness goals. What you eat just has such a powerful impact on your body and health!

It was one of the happiest times in my life: I was pushing myself physically and mentally and loving every minute of it!

I feel truly privileged to have worked alongside Geoff and Andrew and learnt from them on a daily basis. I couldn't have asked for a better grounding in the fitness world and I am so thankful to Andrew and Geoff for giving me that opportunity.

During my time at Vision my life took another unexpected turn, when this big guy called John Beach walked in one day and said that he wanted to start training. He had broken his hand playing soccer and, with his cast finally off, he needed to get back into shape. We hit it off straight away and I really enjoyed training him, but from my perspective, at that time, there was nothing more there than the normal client–trainer relationship.

I thought John was a great guy and he always made me laugh. Then, one fateful Valentine's Day, two dozen red roses and an anonymous poem were delivered to my work. What can I say? The rest is history! He proposed to me on top of The Remarkables in Queenstown, New Zealand, and we married in March 2004. We have two beautiful young children together, Wesley and Chelsea, and we couldn't be happier!

I decided to take some time away from working life while I was having our kids. John travels a lot with his job and the thought of juggling personal training work and the daily routine of two young children seemed nearly impossible. Ironically, I actually called on Mr Smith's advice again for a short time when I took up an at-home admin role with my brother's freight and distribution business.

At the time I didn't know it, but I was about to enter one of the toughest periods of my life. If you've had young kids and struggled to balance work and household commitments, then chances are you totally get where I was coming from. The lack of sleep mixed with the demands of a young family and work commitments made me feel like a zombie most of the time.

I was lucky that I could work from home but that also meant I wasn't getting out of the house very much, which definitely had an effect on my mental state at the time. It didn't help that Wesley wasn't a great sleeper and I would often find myself spending the whole day in my pyjamas and never leaving our apartment, especially if John was away.

I was giving everything I had to balancing my work and family commitments. At the end of the day, I had nothing left emotionally to give to myself. This experience taught me two valuable life lessons: firstly, the importance of exercise and nutrition to keeping a healthy and positive state of mind; and secondly, even when times are at their toughest, you have to make yourself a priority, by taking some time out to focus on 'you'.

As the kids got older, life started to regain some sense of normality and slowly but surely I was finding my mojo again. I quit my office administration career for the second and last time (thank you, Mr Smith) and started training again regularly. The fog had finally lifted and I was ready to jump back into the health and fitness industry.

For the first time in a long while, I was feeling great, getting plenty of sleep and really enjoying life with my loving family! But I had an urge to find a way to make a difference in the world that just wouldn't go away. I knew that something big was on the horizon, I just wasn't sure exactly what it was or how I could make it happen.

HOW IT ALL STARTED

Everything became clear to me just after Christmas 2013.

It was a stunning Sydney day and John and I were able to go for a long afternoon walk; my mother-in-law was in town and looked after the kids for a few hours. It is safe to say that that walk changed the direction of my life forever!

Apart from my formal study, I had spent years immersing myself in health, nutrition and fitness and I knew that I needed to find an outlet to share my passion with like-minded women everywhere. I was constantly being asked by friends and people I knew about how to train and what to eat. With so much misinformation out there and so many quick-fix diets on the market, I knew that my philosophy around training and eating was going to simplify things and make it easier for people to understand.

I especially wanted my philosophy to resonate with busy mums in a similar position, who are constantly being bombarded by shake diets, hormone drops and other short-term, unsustainable health and weight-loss solutions that are advertised on TV and in magazines.

Around that time, social media was really starting to explode and as we walked, John and I talked about what I planned to do with my big dreams. When we got home, we put together a basic plan and strategy for a new Facebook page and blog called Kim Beach Fit Fun Fabulous. This was going to be specifically targeted at busy women and mums all over Australia and – eventually and hopefully – the world!

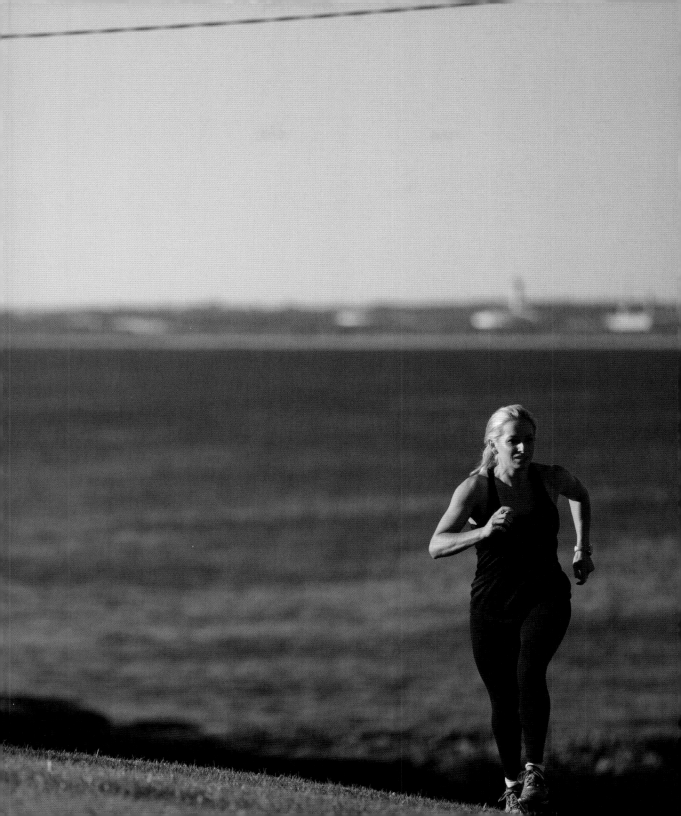

I remember coming back from that walk so excited that I felt like I was going to burst! For the first time in ages, I was going to do something that would enable me to utilise my life's passion and perhaps one day turn it into a full-time job that could positively impact on the lives of others.

Two weeks later – after lots of scribbling in notebooks and late-night planning sessions – I launched my Facebook page with a post about what I had eaten for breakfast that morning. I remember the first few weeks being a real roller-coaster of emotions, as I was putting myself and my ideas out there to the world. I guess there is a small part of everyone that gets a little worried about how people will react and what others might think of them?

That being said, I was absolutely delighted with all the positive comments I was getting from people, which far outweighed any negative thoughts in my head. Day after day my Facebook 'likes' were increasing and I was becoming more and more confident as people were engaging with and reacting to my posts.

By about July of that year, I had more than 35,000 Facebook followers and it was obvious that my message was really starting to be heard. It was then that I knew I had the foundation to create something really special, which is when things started to ramp up.

Like any business I needed money to grow, but the problem was I didn't have anything to sell or any revenue. This issue resulted in a pretty intense conversation between John and me about whether or not we were going to put all the money and resources we had into my new venture. This kind of move doesn't come cheaply.

After much heated back-and-forth discussion, I ended up yelling: 'I JUST WANT TO HELP PEOPLE!' That was the moment I really felt I had found my true purpose and I knew that John could feel it too, because he agreed to risk everything to support me and my new venture. Looking back now, I know that he just needed to clarify whether or not this was something that was going to become my life's work, or just a hobby or part-time job to bring in some extra money.

The next 12 months were a real leap of faith as I continued to invest money in building my venture with very little money coming in.

In my head, I wanted to create some unique training and nutrition programs that were simple to follow, offered genuine support and were affordable for women everywhere. It had taken me years of practical learning and research but I knew I had a philosophy that would work. I just had to make it easy to access online and share in a way that was simple to understand.

It had been a few years since I had put people through their paces in the gym, so I wanted to start the process by working one-on-one with a small number of women to refine my ideas. So I started posting and letting my followers know about my one-on-one program: I ended up working with 12 inspiring women and was able to help them get into a fantastic rhythm with their food and training and, most importantly, help them achieve great results.

After going through the one-on-one process with these amazing women I was so excited, as I knew there was a need for what I was doing. This is when my eight-week online #noexcuses and #nolimits programs were born. The number of visitors to my website was continually growing and tens of thousands of women were downloading my free recipes every month.

Fast-forward to the present and it completely blows my mind that I have several hundred thousand followers on social media. More than 250,000 people are visiting my website every month and I have an amazing team of people around me who help me share my philosophy and programs with the world.

Things are certainly a bit different today from when I took that walk in early 2013, but my message is still the same. It's all about training hard, eating well and living a fitter, healthier life. This book will explain how you can achieve this in a simple yet practical way that can become part of your life forever.

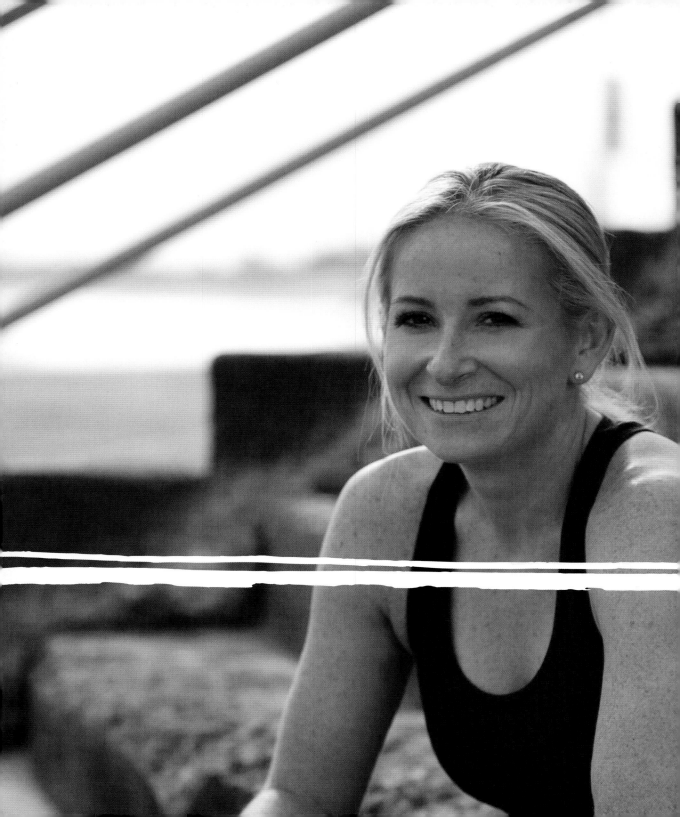

MY PHILOSOPHY OF NUTRITION AND TRAINING

Chapter 1

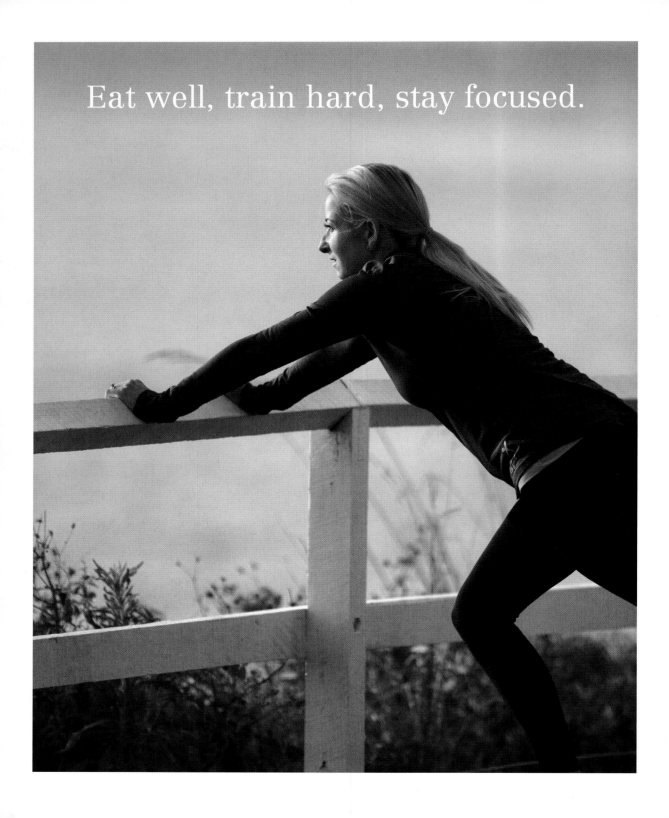

Above all else, I believe in fuelling your body with what I call 'real food', regardless of whether you want to lose weight, change your body shape or just feel fitter and stronger. Eighty per cent of the way to achieve these goals is going to come down to what you eat.

The fitness industry has sold us the idea, for way too long, that the answer to perfect health or an amazing body can be found on a cross-trainer, a treadmill or in a group exercise class. The reality is that, while training is important, it is what you put in your mouth every day that is going to make the critical difference to how you look and – more importantly – how you feel.

I constantly get asked about the training side of my programs but it isn't until people start to see results that they see that the hard work is done in the kitchen – not in your new active wear!

When I say 'real food', what I mean is foods that are not processed, modified or come from a packet. I am talking about vegetables, fruit, lean meats and whole grains. Your body is going to be able to process them efficiently and use them for fuel. You will also find yourself feeling better and having a lot more energy every day. I call my philosophy 'Positive Nutrition': it is the way I choose to live my life on a daily basis.

The second cornerstone of my philosophy is what I call my '80:20 Rule', which is really about focusing on consistency rather than perfection. Let's face it, we are not machines and we can't just eat and drink perfectly every day of our lives. There will always be events to attend, plans to catch up with friends and moments when we just want to let our hair down and enjoy ourselves.

The key is to keep this in balance and aim to fuel your body with real food 80 per cent of the time. I think the biggest mistake you can make is adopting the 'all or nothing' approach, where you are either 100 per cent on point with your eating and training, or completely off and it's back to wine and cheese five nights a week! I will deal with this subject in more detail later on in the book, but it is really important not to put pressure on yourself to be perfect all of the time and to allow yourself to go out and have fun without any feelings of guilt or anxiety. You have to create your own balance between looking after yourself consistently and allowing yourself to indulge and enjoy some treats 20 per cent of the time.

The way you train your body is also a key part of living a fitter, healthier life. I like to use the word 'train' rather than 'exercise', as I think it is more powerful and it implies that you have purpose in what you are doing, with a firm goal in mind. My training philosophy is similar to my philosophy around eating: I believe in embracing all different kinds of training as part of a practical ongoing regime. As with diet, there will always be people telling you that a particular way of doing something is the only way you will achieve results. I disagree with this and believe that adopting all forms of training – in the same way as embracing all major food groups – will help you sustain your results over time.

Having said this, one type of training that I am really passionate about, especially for women, is weight training. It is a must-do for all women, as the benefits are incredible across the board. Weight training will give you shape, it will make you stronger and, best of all, it will help you burn fat all day long. I know it is easy to be intimidated at the thought of weight training, particularly at the gym, so later in this book I will teach you a simple way to get into weight training that you can do just about anywhere. I do weight training three times a week and it is one part of my routine that I just couldn't live without.

When it comes to cardio, I believe in incorporating both High Intensity Interval Training (HIIT) and longer cardio sessions into your training week. HIIT sessions are great for me as I can get them done inside 20 minutes – and I can do them anywhere – which means there are no excuses when it comes to fitting them into my busy days. Longer cardio sessions can be anything from taking the dog for a brisk walk to a nice long run.

Everyone will be at a different stage of fitness and success is all about setting your expectations at the right level and not comparing your journey to anyone else's. This is another trap you can fall into. When you start comparing yourself to other people you will never be happy, as there will always be someone who is fitter, faster or stronger than you. The key is to focus on your own journey, measure your own progress and don't forget to celebrate your successes along the way!

As you have probably gathered by now, my philosophy focuses on the long term, not overnight promises. If there is one thing that gets my blood boiling it is the quick-fix diet and exercise industry. I think the general public are slowly starting to wake up to the fact that these short-term solutions don't work. It amazes me how many products I still see promising to give you unbelievable results in just a few days or weeks. I guess as humans we want to believe that this is possible, which is why we buy them, but let's be honest with one another: has anyone ever bought an abs machine or switched to meal-replacement shakes and actually seen long-term results? The same can be said for diet pills, detox diets, calorie restriction or hormone products. I have yet to meet someone who was actually able to change their body composition and sustain their results using any of these fads or quick fixes.

I promise you that the long-term solution for a fitter and healthier lifestyle is based around eating well, training hard, staying consistent and, most of all, enjoying your journey.

'Life isn't about finding yourself,
it's about creating yourself.'

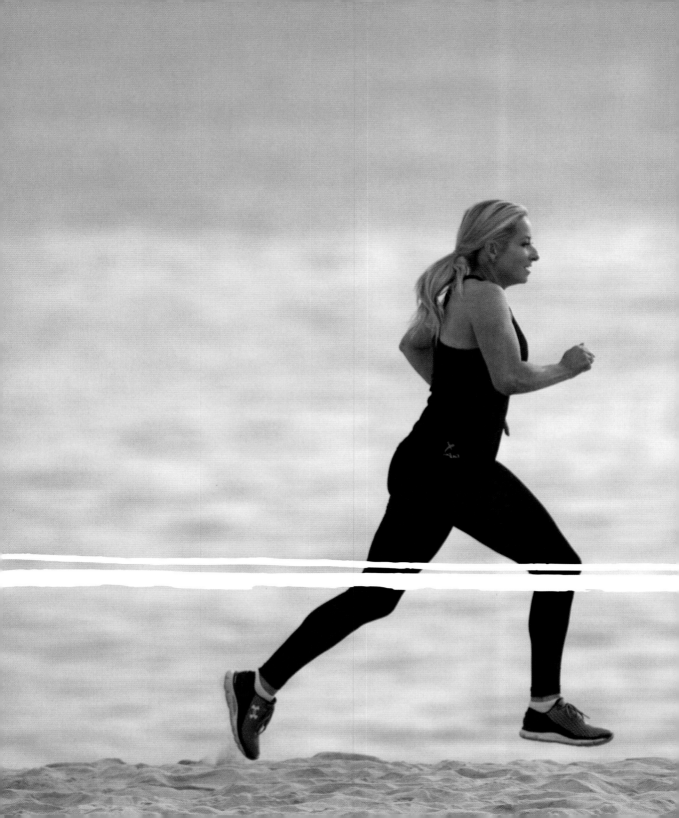

PREPARING FOR SUCCESS

Chapter 2

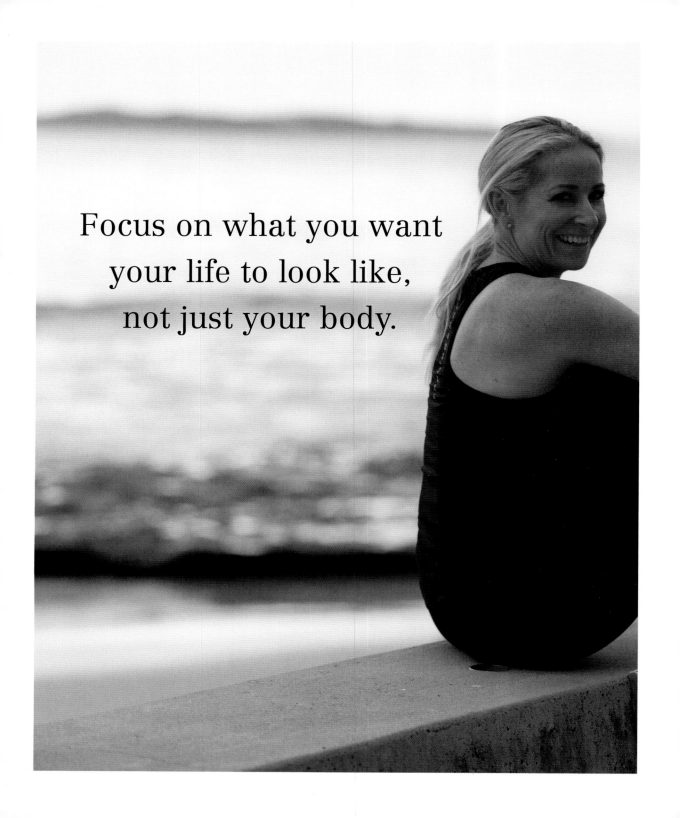

Focus on what you want
your life to look like,
not just your body.

SETTING THE RIGHT GOALS

Whether your goal is weight loss or just living a healthier and fitter life, you need to set clear and firm goals for what you want to achieve. I also suggest you write these down and keep them close to you, so that you see them every day.

Personally, I write them on A3-size pieces of paper and put them up all over my kitchen wall. I am sure the visitors to my house think it's 'a little different', but having the pages staring at me every day keeps me focused on exactly what I want to achieve and how I am going to get there.

Lots of women on my programs have created their own vision boards to help them with this process. I guess it comes down to whether you like pictures or words; however, the key is to keep them visible, so that you can be reminded daily of your goals.

There is real power in writing down your goals: I believe it changes things from just being an idea to being a firm commitment that you need to act upon.

For me, this has been proven to work time and time again, as I tend to reset my kitchen-wall goals every six months – when it's time to take them down and put up new ones, more often than not all the big important ones have been ticked off or even exceeded!

Don't feel weird or embarrassed about writing your goals down or putting them out there. I promise you that some of the most successful people in the world follow this exact process and it has a huge impact on helping them achieve their goals. So, if you can do this right now, please go grab some paper and a pen, make yourself a nice cup of herbal tea and take some time to think about what you really want in life. Write it all down and put it somewhere you can see it every day.

When setting your goals it is important to break them down into small, achievable chunks. For example, if your goal is to lose 30 kilograms then writing down 'I want to lose 30 kilograms' is a great start, but you are going to need to set some smaller goals along the way as these will help you achieve your overall big goal. In this instance your smaller goals could be:

- I will walk three times a week for the next two weeks.

- I will not drink alcohol for the next two weeks.

- I will focus on eating portion-controlled meals full of 'real food' for the next two weeks.

- At the end of two weeks I will feel better, have more energy, sleep better and be ready to take on the next two weeks of goals.

Setting a shorter time limit for smaller goals is vital and you need to make them easily achievable. In this instance, I have used two weeks as a time frame, as it is quite possible to stay away from alcohol and focus on eating well for that period.

If you continue to repeat this process, you will find that you can start to extend the time frames and also add some actual goals for weight loss; however, I strongly suggest that if weight loss is your goal, you only actually weigh yourself every four weeks to get a true reading on your progress and avoid the day-to-day roller-coaster ride the scales often provide. Even better, if you are up for the challenge, put your scales away for good and don't include them as part of your journey. Instead, focus purely on how you feel and how your clothes fit you. I talk about this in more detail on page 33.

It is exactly the same process if your big goal is to run a half marathon. You need to break this down into smaller, more manageable goals; in this example, your smaller goals could be based around being able to run for half an hour without stopping (depending on your level of fitness, of course) or making sure you get eight hours' sleep a night before your morning run four times per week. The key again is setting a firm time frame for each goal and making the goal real and achievable, based on where you are at today.

Remember that all your small goals should feed into your bigger goal and I would suggest setting between two and four goals for any given two-week period. It can also help to have a specific time and day, such as a Saturday afternoon when you are not too busy, when you can take the time to reset your goals and reflect on what you have achieved. Don't forget to celebrate your progress, as enjoying your journey is a critical aspect to success in the long term.

I also suggest you share your goals, both big and small, with those closest to you. Just as putting them out into the universe has power, so does sharing them with the people you love and trust. There are going to be times along the way when you doubt yourself and your ability to get things done. This is where having a trusted support crew comes into play, as they tend to have a unique way of reminding you of how amazing you actually are – and why you set your goals in the first place!

There is also a lot of benefit in setting a crazy, scary, long-term goal and it is something that you should definitely do. This needs to be bigger and scarier than your 'lose 30kg' or 'run a half marathon' goal. For this one, you might need to close your eyes and really focus on how you see yourself and what you really want to achieve in your life. Once you can put your finger on this, it will provide you with a clear path and genuine clarity in relation to all your other goals. Write it down and get it up on the wall!

My big, scary, crazy goal is about using the power of my business and our global #beachfit community to help women in need around the world lead fitter, healthier lives. This is always in the back of my mind as I'm working through my shorter-term goals; I even have this crazy dream of one day talking to Ellen DeGeneres about this live on her television show!

I use the word 'scary' as I believe this goal has to really scare you and seem almost impossible. This way it will push your boundaries, stretch your mind and really get you thinking about what might be possible in your life.

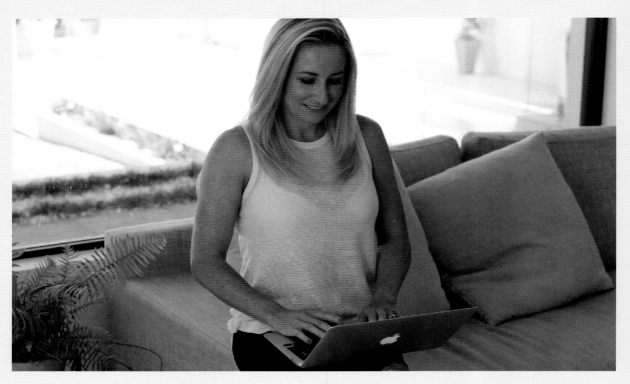

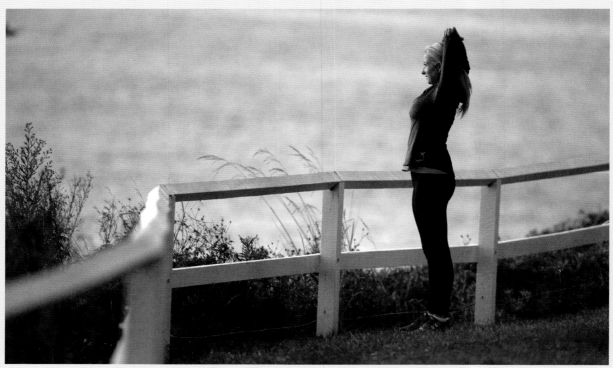

BEING ORGANISED!

Being properly organised is one of the real keys to making your health-and-fitness journey a success. You can have all the right intentions, but it is preparation and creating the right habits that will be the difference between success and failure in the long run.

This organisation and preparation falls into two key areas:

1. Scheduling your training sessions every week.
2. Planning your food for the week ahead.

I tend to be totally flat out with work and family commitments during the week, so I choose to take a few hours on a Sunday afternoon to make sure I have ticked off these two important points. I do this religiously every week and it sets me up for a great seven days ahead.

My training gets scheduled into my calendar each week. I try to do a minimum of three weights and two cardio sessions every week. It doesn't matter what type of sessions you are doing, as this will relate to your own goals; the key is to get them locked in and mentally commit to them ahead of time.

Planning ahead like this also means there is less chance something will come up at the last minute that will prevent you from doing your sessions. As busy women, I understand that we tend to prioritise work and family commitments, but you have to make time for yourself and scheduling your training sessions is one of the best ways to ensure you do this.

It's amazing how refreshed and energised you can feel, both mentally and physically, after even a short walk, run or weights session.

Even more important than scheduling your training sessions is the planning and preparing of your food for the week ahead. I don't know what it is like at your place, but for me it is all about enjoying a simple, nutritious family meal every night. I just don't have the time or the energy to produce a gourmet masterpiece on demand for my family on weeknights. John is often either away for work or gets home after 6pm, which means that I need to be organised ahead of time.

What I also find is that a lack of preparation with your food can quickly translate into fish and chips, pizza or burgers, when time and effort are big factors in your meal choice on any given night. This type of behaviour probably won't help you to achieve any of the important goals that you have written down and set for yourself.

In practical terms, this means I will prepare something like the following on a Sunday afternoon.

CHOC MINT PROTEIN BALLS (SEE RECIPE, PAGE 185)

Super-easy to make and store in the fridge. These are my go-to treats for the week and are wonderful with a green tea.

SWEET POTATO DEVILLED EGGS (SEE RECIPE, PAGE 141)

This is my favourite choice for Meal 2, which I eat around 10am each day. I generally boil up six eggs at a time, which lasts me for three days.

CHICKEN AND QUINOA MEATLOAF (SEE RECIPE, PAGE 155)

This recipe is a complete winner for lunch and actually tastes better two or three days after you make it, as the flavours intensify. You can freeze it or store it in the fridge for a few days.

TUNA AND SWEET POTATO PATTIES (SEE RECIPE, PAGE 149)

Another perfect pre-made lunch option; you can also eat these cold and they taste AMAZING!

PORK SAN CHOY BAU (SEE RECIPE, PAGE 173)

This is by far the most popular recipe in my 8-week program. This is ideal for dinner and I promise your whole family will love it!

BROWN RICE AND QUINOA

I usually cook up a cup of each, let them cool, then store them in an airtight container in the fridge. Having these all ready to go in the fridge makes it so much easier to create meals like my Sweet Mustard Chicken Salad (see recipe, page 147) or Turkey Wrap (see recipe, page 144).

During the course of reading this book, you will probably hear me talking frequently about 'consistency'. Being organised is vital and achieving this consistently every week will create a new habit that will become beneficial in the long term.

Everything that I have outlined above is what I do every Sunday without fail. This means that sometimes I have to sacrifice other things – usually social activities or catching up with my favourite TV shows – in order to be in a position to realise my long-term goals; however, over time you learn from experience and are able to do things more quickly and efficiently, so you can spend time doing the things that you want to do. I believe these small sacrifices are totally worth it, as feeling healthy and strong will always be more important to me than knowing who made the final four in a reality TV show.

So, now your training is all organised and your food is prepped, we need to talk about the all-important 'S word' …

'Strength doesn't come from what you can do, it comes from overcoming the things that you once thought you couldn't.'

SLEEP

Getting the right amount of sleep on a regular basis will give you the energy you need to train hard, stay mentally focused and keep working towards your goals. On the flip side, not getting the required amount of sleep will make you cranky, unorganised (probably skipping training sessions and meals) and have you reaching for the nearest chocolate bar as you do your last-minute dash to the supermarket.

I cannot emphasise enough how important sleep is when it comes to staying focused and positive on a daily basis. If you are the mother of young kids and you're reading this right now, you're probably thinking, 'What the hell is sleep?!', which I totally understand: my son was awake every 2–3 hours for the first three years of my parenthood experience. If this sounds like you, then please know that things will improve as time goes on and just for now take whatever time out and rest you can get. For everyone else, please start prioritising between 6–8 hours of quality sleep a night.

I like to get up at 5am every day. It provides me with a little bit of 'me' time every morning to get my head straight for the day. Also I like to knock off at least an hour's work before my kids jump out of bed and the fun starts.

For me this means getting to bed by 10pm every night as I need at least a solid 6–8 hours rest to operate effectively. Everyone is different and it might take you some time to adjust to doing this, but if you are training hard and eating well I promise your body will get used to it really quickly. The weekends are obviously a little different with social and family events, but I always feel amazing if I have had solid sleeps Sunday through to Thursday.

Taking the time each week to plan your food and training will be one of the most important factors when it comes to realising your weight loss and health-and-fitness goals. Throw in 6–8 hours of quality sleep five days a week and you should start to see the results you want!

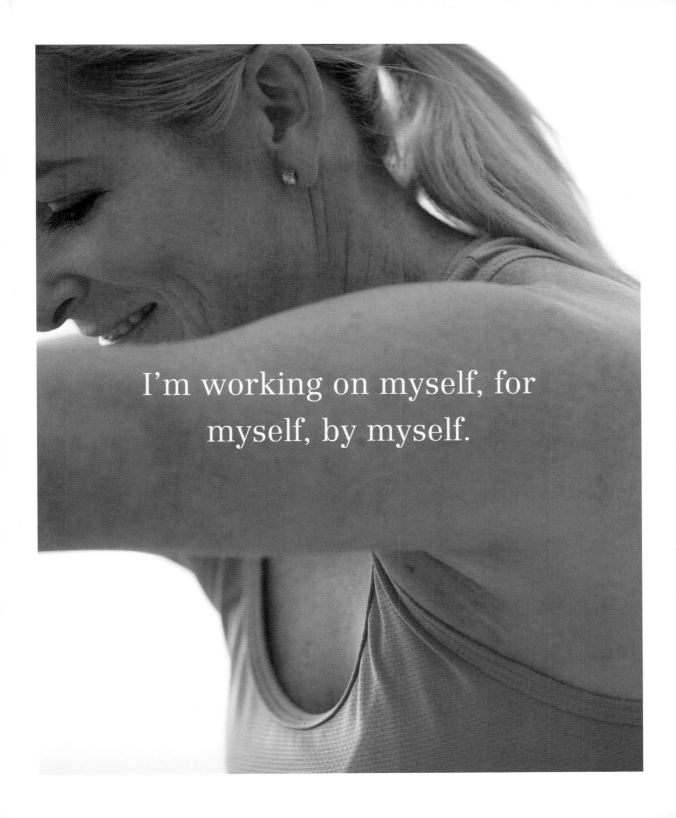

ALL OR NOTHING: IT'S TIME TO STOP!

Do you struggle with sticking to a new health regime for more than a few weeks? Or maybe you find yourself saying, 'Okay, I will just start again next Monday'? If this sounds like you, then this chapter has been written especially with you in mind. I mentioned this subject in the introduction: the 'all or nothing' approach, when it comes to weight loss, health and fitness has to STOP NOW!

This approach simply encourages a nasty, vicious cycle of 'yo-yo' dieting and consistent feelings of guilt and failure. I have designed weight-loss programs that are eight weeks long but they are written specifically to prepare you for a long-term change in lifestyle. This is also the reason why I spent a lot of time creating a specific program to help people transitioning from a 100 per cent weight-loss phase back into a healthy life and routine.

A lifestyle change – or just wanting to become healthier – should not come with a beginning and an end date. Most people have a fantastic reason for wanting to make positive changes in their lives. These include wanting to live longer, to minimise the chance of disease and to be able to spend more quality time with their family and children. These are reasons that require a long-term change in mindset and thinking. No one says, 'I want to spend more quality time with my children for the next 12 weeks,' so why is it okay that they would only commit to training hard and eating well for a short period of time?

I think one of the reasons it can be hard to mentally adjust to this way of thinking is the fear of failure. How many times have you tried some new way of eating, only to go out for dinner on a Wednesday night, overindulge and then think, 'I've wrecked it all now, so I might as well just reset the clock next week.' You didn't wreck it; it's called 'life' and unless you are going to lock yourself in a room for the next 40 years, you will have to get used to enjoying social situations as part of a positive lifestyle change!

I often see in my programs that some women get to day 14 or 15 and have a bad day or weekend, for whatever reason. They then think that the best solution is to go back to day 1. This drives me crazy! This is just normal life! Stay focused, look forward and put all your energy into the week ahead, so you can continue to maintain your new healthy habits. Beating yourself up about not being perfect will do nothing other than make you feel like a failure time and time again.

This is what my 80:20 rule is all about; once you start to enjoy eating 'real food' and realise the positive effect it has on the way you feel, the less likely you are to make poor nutritional choices. You will also learn to really enjoy those times when you do go out for a great meal and a few drinks, without the feeling of guilt. Sure, you may force yourself to go to a double spin class the next day, but you will be happy knowing that 80 per cent of the time you're training hard and fuelling your body correctly.

This is my philosophy and it works for me, but it did take years of trial and error to finally understand that a healthy lifestyle is all about consistency, not perfection. Recently, one client told me, 'I'm not always 100 per cent, but I have a lot of 100 per cent days!' She is bang on the money! Enjoy the times when you are eating and training consistently and also enjoy the times when you get to cut loose for a little bit.

A great way to ensure you can successfully throw the 'all or nothing' theory out the window is to throw your bathroom scales out along with it. There are simply too many factors that can affect the number between your feet every day. It is crazy to let scales dictate your emotions.

For example, let's say it's early in your journey and you have put all your effort into a great week of eating and exercise. You are feeling great, sleeping well and you have tons more energy. Then, you jump on the scales and it is the same number as it was a week ago. What happens next is usually classic self-sabotage, where you follow up a week of positive effort with a glass of wine or some chocolate, thinking, 'What's the point?' Please do yourself a favour and throw your scales away, or at least put them high up in a cupboard somewhere. Judge your progress first and foremost by the way you feel and secondly by the way your clothes fit and the changes to your body that you can see in the mirror.

The other thing to keep in mind, at the start of any journey, is that it may take up to four weeks for your body to figure out what the hell is going on. You could feel lethargic, light-headed and just downright awful, but this is your body ridding itself of all the accumulated toxins and is to be expected. Please consult your doctor if you are worried about any ongoing symptoms.

Just keep making good decisions and if you do happen to find yourself on the wrong side of a serving of hot chips, then know that it is okay and don't feel guilty. You didn't fail, you are human and it will happen from time to time, probably for the rest of your life. Try not to think about the sick feeling that the hot chips probably gave you and put all your focus and energy into your next meal, your next day and your next training session.

If any of this section resonates with you, please stop and have a serious think about changing your approach to eating and training. Be prepared to focus on doing the right things, but be kind to yourself and know that perfection is an impossible standard to achieve. You are human after all.

'It's not about being perfect. It's about effort: when you bring that effort every single day, that's when change happens.'

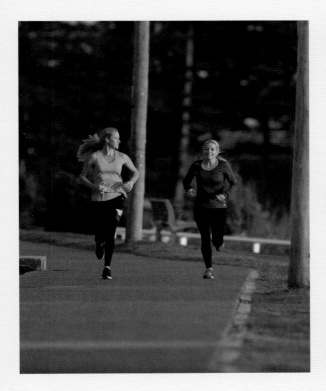
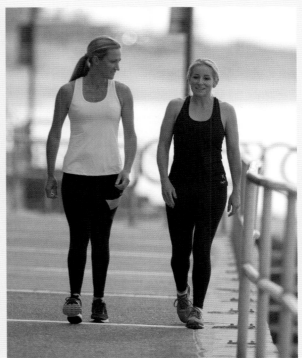
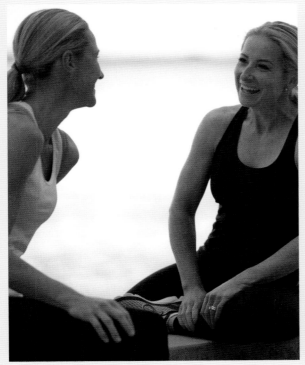
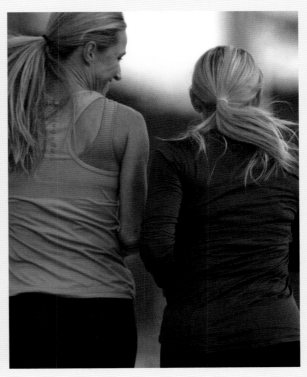

YOUR CIRCLE OF INFLUENCE

I spend my professional life helping women lose weight sustainably and teaching them how to create and maintain fitter, healthier lifestyles. This is one of the most rewarding things anyone can do, but it never ceases to amaze me how negative some people can be towards these inspiring women who want to make a positive change in their lives. I constantly see and hear stories about women trying really hard to create positive change, who are then pulled down by people around them, instead of being encouraged and supported along their journey.

One classic example came from a woman – let's call her Sarah – who had achieved a ten kilogram weight loss on my #noexcuses program and was well on track to achieving her goals. Sarah was an active member of my private online support group and was always positive and encouraging other women on the program. At this point, Sarah was probably a size 14–16 and, in her words, still had some way to go to achieve her ultimate goal. Her confidence after eight weeks was sky high, based on the results she had achieved and the progress she was making.

Sarah bought a new dress and was out to dinner with some friends, having an amazing night and feeling fantastic about herself. She got up to go to the toilet and as she was returning to the table she overheard one of her friends laughing and remarking, 'Well, she's still fat!'

I cannot imagine how Sarah must have felt at this point in time. She was eight weeks into her new lifestyle change, had lost ten kilograms and was finally starting to feel like a new version of herself, only to be put down by one of her so-called friends in a disgusting way that I can only describe as bullying.

When I heard about this I was SO angry at the potential damage that such a thoughtless comment could do. It could easily have led to Sarah undoing all her hard work. Sarah was just two months into a new lifestyle, feeling on top of the world and she was going to continue her journey of weight loss with vigour ... and to think that it could have all come undone just because of one pathetic comment!

I can't even comprehend the mindset of this other woman but I know I feel extremely sorry for her. Maybe she isn't totally confident in her own life and attacking Sarah in this way was a way to cope? Who knows?

Fortunately for Sarah, she was part of my amazing online #noexcuses community. So, when she posted about this incident in the support group she literally had hundreds of women going into bat for her and telling her exactly what they thought of her friend's comments, reminding her that she had already achieved something amazing and it wasn't over yet.

The point of this story is to show you that the people you choose to surround yourself with could be the difference between successfully making the changes you want and being made to feel like a failure. Sarah's example was one of the worst I have seen, but I have heard many other stories, particularly within families, where people would rather see someone dragged down to their level than focus on helping them make progress on their journey of change.

If you are part of a family or network of friends who don't share your interests in a healthier lifestyle, you really need to sit down with them individually and talk about the changes you are looking to make and why. Ask them for their support and, hopefully, you will receive it, as they come to understand your reasons for wanting to change. Who knows – you may even inspire them to join you.

One of the hardest things in life is to stay unaffected by what people say around you. I think it stems back to when we were all subjected to some form of teasing at school and the most important thing at the time was to have the favour of your classmates. Unfortunately, this mentality is often not left behind in the schoolyard and can be carried on in your day-to-day life as an adult.

I have personally made a conscious decision not to participate in this behaviour in my life and I encourage you to do the same. Sure, it's meant that my circle of friends has changed over the years, but now I choose to surround myself with positive people who want to help me achieve my goals and in turn I give them 100 per cent of my love, support and commitment. Life's too short to spend time and energy talking about or putting down other people. Wouldn't the world be a better place if we all consciously chose to do the opposite?

The bottom line is, if you want to make a positive change in your life when it comes to health and fitness, then you have to make sure that you have people around you who are going to support your efforts and be a significant part of your journey.

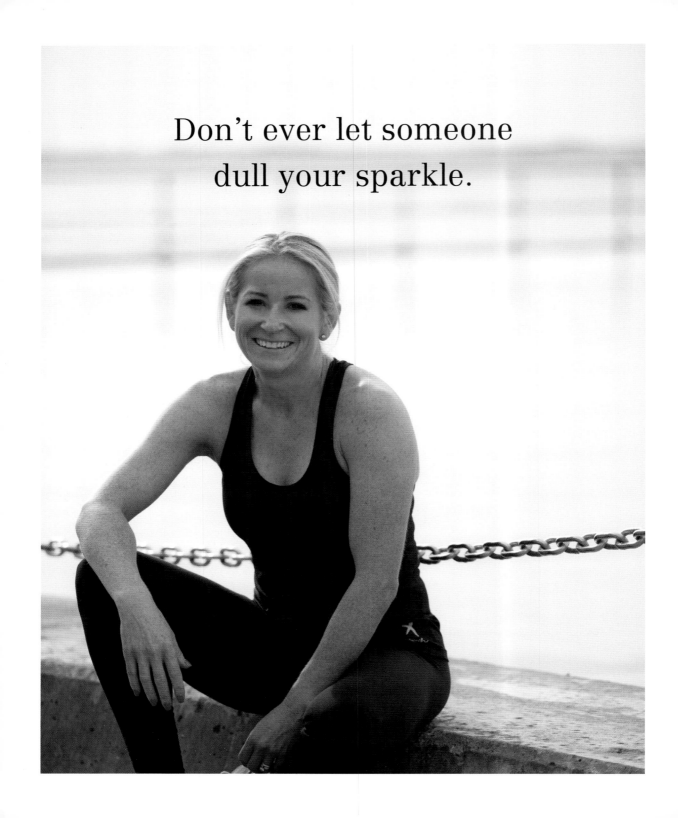

Don't ever let someone
dull your sparkle.

SIMPLE IS BEST

In 2013, my big scary goal was to compete in an International Natural Bodybuilding Association (INBA) body-building competition. There are two main reasons I wanted to do this: firstly, I just wanted to see if I could get my body into that shape after giving birth to two kids; and, secondly, I wanted to test some of my training and nutrition theories on reducing body fat – there was no better person to use as a guinea pig than myself!

I take my hat off to any woman or man who gets up on that stage. I totally respect and appreciate the absolute commitment, focus and hard work required to get your body stage ready. Having said this, it is something I will NEVER do again. I enjoyed many aspects of the preparation and training, but getting up on stage was definitely not for me. This became brutally evident when I almost fell over, not once but twice, in front of the judges at a national event in Melbourne. Heels and sparkly bikinis are definitely not my thing!

On a serious note, I found that as I got closer to the event I started to obsess more and more about my food and training. It consumed my whole life and not in a positive way. The crunch moment was when my son Wesley, who was six at the time, turned around to me and said, 'When will my normal mummy be back?'

I had let my pursuit of health and fitness overtake some of the other very important things in my life. This made me realise how important balance is and that consistency is much better then aiming for perfection.

Any successful lifestyle change requires balance and is best kept simple. Your normal routine will probably change for the better, but you can't go from being all one way to all the other and expect to sustain this over time. I see this behaviour a lot in the women I work with, when they will obsess over small things that really don't make much difference at the end of the day.

Whether you are doing a 20-kilogram bench press or a 30-kilogram bench press doesn't matter: you are still lifting weights, which is the important thing. The same goes for food: whether you are having 100 grams of chicken or 150 grams of chicken really doesn't matter, it is just great that you are eating a lean protein that will aid in building muscle instead of all the other unhealthy options you might normally be consuming.

This is particularly important if you are starting a lifestyle change, where you need to focus on just doing the right things, rather than obsessing and getting lost in all the detail. On the other hand, if you are training for a specific purpose or event, then the details may become more important.

You also need to realise that there can be more than one speed to your efforts. It is perfectly normal to want to start anything new at absolute top speed, as you are going to be really motivated and full of enthusiasm. Just as when you are driving a car and you need to slow down and change gears occasionally, that doesn't mean you need to stop the car and pull over completely.

For example, as I am writing this book, my training at the moment is down to two sessions a week. I am currently running in second gear with my training and that is okay, because it is just a matter of time before I accelerate into fourth and fifth gears again. There will be times in your life when you will come up against a red light and you will need to stop and restart. Just know that you still have all those gears available to you and you can't use them all at once.

Unfortunately, technology isn't helping my 'keep it simple' philosophy, as every step and kilojoule can now be counted by your smart phone or smart watch and this provides another opportunity for you to obsess over a number that, in the grand scheme of things, won't dictate your success or failure.

On the very rare occasion that I do a spin class, the bike tells me that I burn somewhere between 1500–2000 kilojoules in 45 minutes. This would be great if I wanted a bike to tell me how I was going, but I would rather rely on the sweat that I left on the floor during the session and knowing how hard I had worked mentally as a way of judging my workout.

You aren't going to set a personal best in every spin class or for every five-kilometre run that you go on, so you need to pay more attention to the fact that you have done the exercise in the first place and enjoy the feeling that you get when those endorphins kick in.

What I am saying is that the people I see succeed in the long term are the ones who have kept it simple and have taken the time to actually enjoy the changes they have made in their lives, rather than obsessing over the details. You need to prepare for a marathon not a sprint! Once you get your head around the fact that there is no beginning or end date to what you are trying to achieve, you will well and truly be on the right path to success.

'You are in control: making the right choices is up to you.'

'If you want the rainbow, sometimes you have to deal with the rain.'

'Positive minds live positive lives.'

CECILIA'S STORY

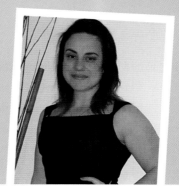

My story is much like many women out there: from a young age my weight has always fluctuated and, like a lot of females, I developed a somewhat unhealthy relationship with the mirror, food and exercise.

In retrospect I hated the way I looked and have had many times where I've reached my goal weight but was unable to maintain it, therefore I settled back into my usual size 14.

I am now a single mother of two beautiful children, and find that I'm always doing things for them and others before myself. A slump in my life saw me take a turn towards depression, having dealt with a volatile marriage then divorce and so on, which led me down an even more unhealthy path. All the previous methods that had worked to shift weight were no longer working for me.

Hair loss, achy muscles, fatigue and weight gain were all symptoms that my thyroid had slowed down. I sought medical advice and my suspicions were confirmed. Although not quite at the levels that needed medication, it was right on the cusp.

The turning point for me came three months ago when I saw a picture of myself on social media. I was disgusted by what I saw and the dread of an impending summer season set off a feeling of desperation. I just knew something had to be done.

I decided to contact Kim and ask what the chances of weight management would be for someone with a sluggish thyroid. I was thrilled to be told that by following her advice, I could lose weight and get myself out of my health rut.

The experience exceeded all my expectations. I saw almost instant results, dropping 2.7 kilograms in the first week. I burst into happy tears because I knew I'd finally found a healthy and sound solution to my crisis.

My energy levels skyrocketed and my weight continually dropped at a steady pace of one kilogram per week until, by the end of the eight weeks I had lost nine kilograms and dropped two dress sizes. I'm currently in week 14 and down eleven kilograms to a healthy size 10 and I'm fitter and healthier than I have been since my teens.

Cecilia

HELEN'S STORY

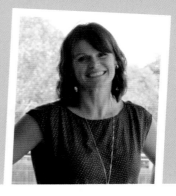

Hi! My name is Helen and I'm a personal trainer. Anybody that I've met over the past two years wouldn't have known that, because I was too embarrassed to say so. My problem was I never felt good enough. I was a damn good personal trainer but I would go to work and compare myself to everyone else. If my clients looked stronger or leaner I thought to myself, 'I should look like that'. Even if the girl was ten years younger than me, even if at the time I was only 63–64 kilos, it was never good enough.

There were a few other contributing factors that helped with the increase of my weight but they were very personal factors and I think I just gave up on myself for a while. I had tried so many diets in the past and, yes, had lost weight with some, but could never keep it off. I always felt like a failure and I was increasingly becoming addicted to sugar, fats and binging on food.

The first thing that attracted me to Kim's program was her philosophy of 'no excuses'. I have in the past used way too many excuses and enough was enough. I so badly wanted to change. Yes I wanted to lose weight but most of all I wanted to change my mindset. I think I finally got to breaking point and I was really ready for change. It was great to be part of an online community with other women going through the same process. The other girls were always on my side and cheering me on, as I did with them.

I got pretty invested in the community, helped a lot of people and advised them on a few things, mostly about getting into the right mindset. This is when I really started to listen to what I was saying. The more comments I gave, the more I was changing in myself. You can't tell someone something and then not take that on board yourself.

I told Kim Beach that I found my 'Holy Grail' when I started on her program. Her advice has changed my whole attitude to my weight, the scales and how I see and respect myself. I have lost a total of 10.4 kilos and still have about 5 kilos to lose. For the first time ever, I know I will get there. Never have I had such faith in myself. I know I'm a changed woman inside and out.

Helen

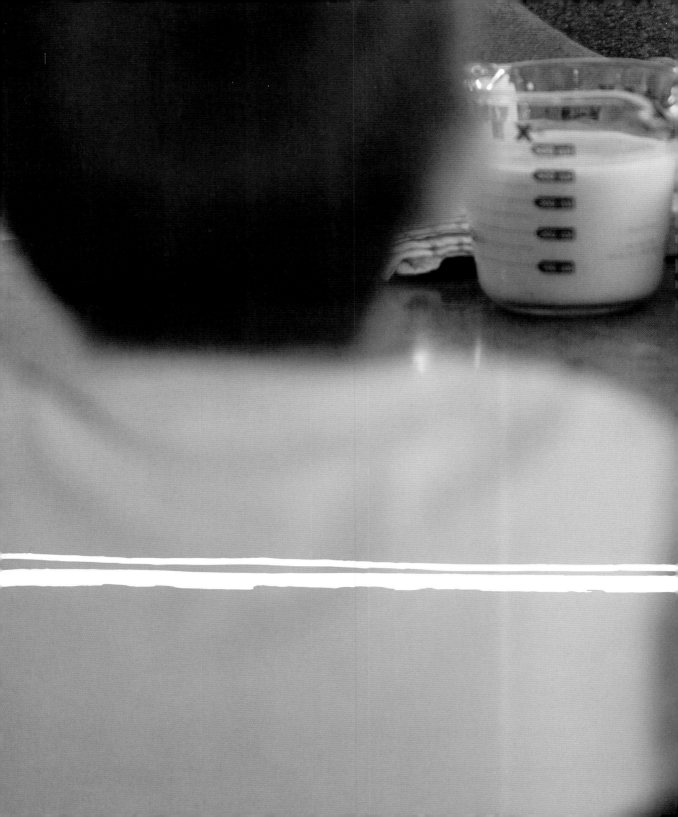

POSITIVE NUTRITION

Chapter 3

Never eat ingredients
you can't pronounce ...
except quinoa.

You should eat quinoa!

WHAT IS POSITIVE NUTRITION?

Proper nutrition is the key to maintaining the weight and body shape you want in the long term. I also believe that eating well can be a huge contributing factor leading to a long and healthy life.

As I mentioned earlier, I don't believe in unsustainable fad diets or any diet that excludes particular food groups. I am also a strong supporter of the fact that you don't need to count calories to get the results that you want, as this process can make you lose focus from your major goal; however, I will speak more to that point later on.

I think it is important to embrace a range of 'real food' as a part of your daily life. I call this **Positive Nutrition**.

My definition of 'real food' is something you eat that hasn't been altered from its original form; for example, fruits, vegetables, nuts, seeds, whole grains and lean cuts of meat. These are all foods that our bodies will recognise and use to nourish themselves correctly.

The other side of this is that I strongly encourage you to steer clear of foods that have been highly processed and hold little to no nutritional value. A quick look at the nutritional panel on any packet will tell you a great deal. Let's face it, most of us can't even pronounce a lot of these ingredients – let alone know what they actually are – but we are happy to put them into our bodies on a daily basis.

There is a reason that all the 'real food' I have mentioned don't have a nutritional panel on the side: they simply don't need one!

In an ideal world, we would all have access to an unlimited range of completely organic produce, so that our decisions would be easy to make. Unfortunately this is not the world that we live in. So, if organic is not an obvious or easy option for you, then you will need to use your common sense and try to buy quality locally sourced produce instead.

One of the major benefits of eating 'real food' is that it can make you feel amazing. A lot of women doing my programs often tell me how great they feel after just a few weeks of eating well. They are more positive, have more energy and find themselves with a higher degree of mental clarity.

I know from personal experience how sluggish and tired I can feel if I overindulge in the wrong foods. If that ever happens, it can take me few days to get back to feeling myself again, both physically and mentally.

When it comes to nutrition, try and keep the 80:20 rule in mind and you can't go too far wrong. It is all about eating the right foods consistently and not focusing on being perfect.

If you eat the right foods consistently, you will get positive long-term results and there should never be any guilt associated with what you are eating. If you do happen to indulge in a packet of chocolate biscuits, don't beat yourself up about it. Just move on and focus on making your next few meals consistently good. Remember, there is no starting or finishing point. This is your life and you need to choose what you put in your mouth every day, as it will dictate your weight and health in the years to come.

SIMPLE, PRACTICAL AND TASTY

One of the cornerstones of my philosophy is that food needs to be tasty, but also needs to be simple. Whether I am making breakfast or a family meal, ideally I want it cooked and served in under 15 minutes. All my recipes are based around this principle and require a minimum of fuss. There is so much to be said for simple cooking methods, as they will retain nutrients in the food. 'Fast food' isn't traditionally associated with being nutritious and healthy, but I promise that there is another side to cooking food quickly that will prove different!

This is why my favourite kitchen appliance is a sandwich press (or toasted sandwich maker), which I use to cook at least three of my meals each day. It is a little ironic that something that was designed to make toasted cheese sandwiches with white bread has become such a focus for my 'real food' philosophy, but trust me when I say that, used the right way, the sandwich press will change your life! If you don't have a sandwich press, you can use a non-stick frying pan instead.

Your weekdays can be absolutely crazy and lacking in time, so in practical terms it is important to do some preparation on the weekend. This means creating a few tasty meals for the week ahead, as well as cooking up some staples, such as quinoa and brown rice, to have ready in the fridge. Remember: preparation is the key to success.

A lot of the tastes we become accustomed to in our food today have been artificially created, something with which I have a real problem. 'Real food' does not mean boring or tasteless. You just need to get creative with your spices and start to experiment more in the kitchen; for example, I will cook chicken, sweet potato and asparagus on the sandwich press for morning tea or lunch and I will always add a spice, such as smoked paprika or curry powder, to add punch and flavour.

Keep it simple, practical and tasty and you can't go wrong!

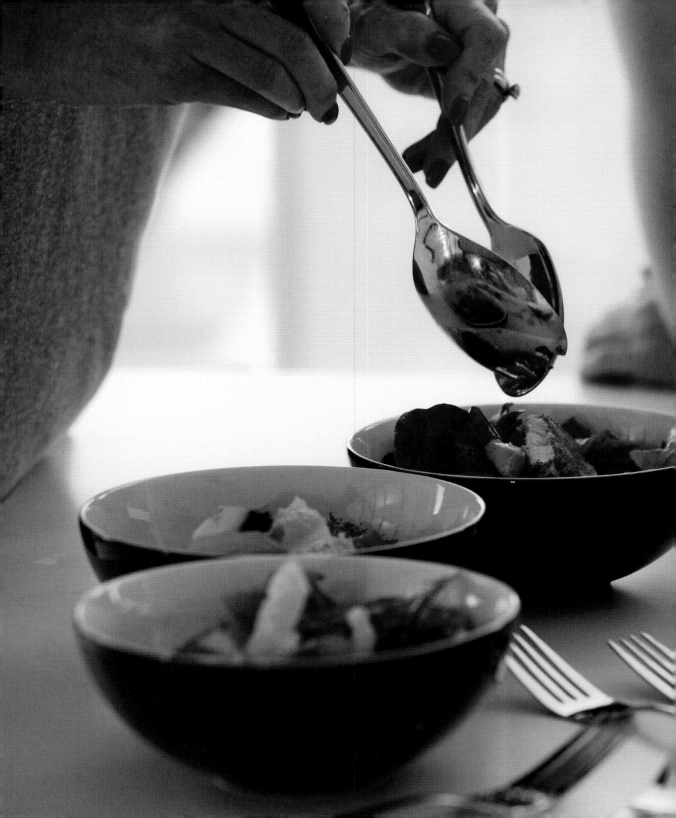

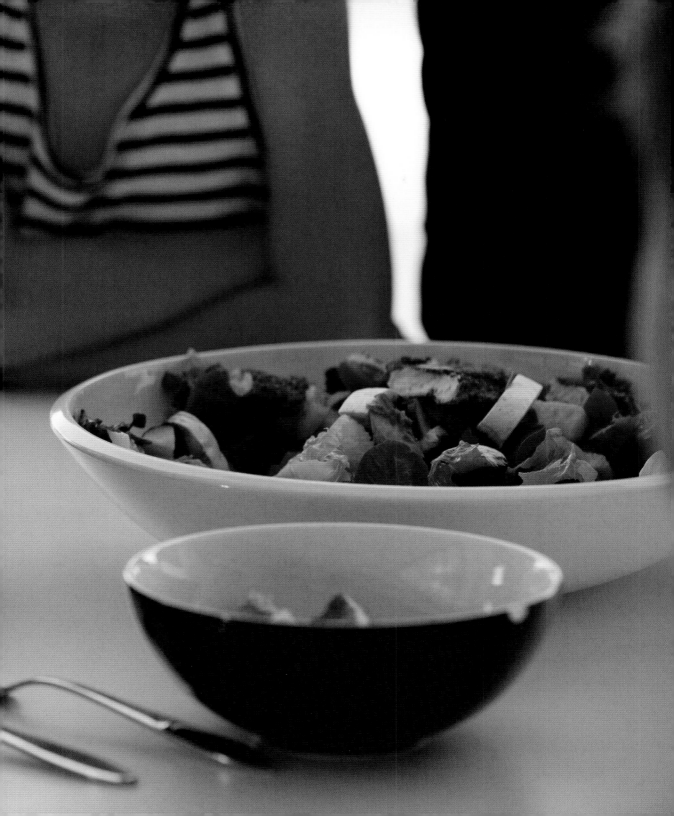

EATING FOR WEIGHT LOSS

Something I am really passionate about is helping people understand the difference between eating to stay healthy and eating for weight loss. There are lots of fantastic healthy foods out there that are great for you, but they won't necessarily help you lose weight. In this section, I talk about the foods that you should be eating to lose weight and discuss which foods to steer clear of.

KEEPING YOUR BLOOD SUGAR STABLE

If weight loss is your goal, then it is vital to keep your blood sugar stable during the course of the day. When you eat food that includes simple sugars, your body reacts by having a high spike in insulin to try to bring your blood sugar levels back to normal. The downside of this is that insulin is a storage hormone, which means there is a very high chance that it will store whatever you are eating as fat. This process is something you definitely want to avoid if you are trying to lose weight.

It is impossible to avoid this process all together, as all foods will affect your blood-sugar level in some way; however, if you focus on eating foods that have a minimal effect on your blood-sugar level then you will give your body the best possible chance to burn fat throughout the day.

The way to achieve this is to focus on carbohydrates that are low GI (Glycaemic Index) and high in fibre, include a small amount of lean protein in every meal and make sure you consume enough good fats every day. All of the recipes in this book adhere to this nutritional philosophy.

I am often asked about cravings. They generally occur when you have a dip in your blood-sugar levels and your body starts to crave the wrong types of foods. A great example of this is if you have had lunch at midday but then eat nothing throughout the afternoon; at about 4pm your body starts screaming for chocolate or something sweet. The way to avoid this is to eat the right type of foods regularly throughout the day.

EATING REGULARLY

I believe in eating regularly throughout the day, with portion size being very important. There are lots of other theories out there and solid arguments to support them, but in my experience nothing replaces eating the right food regularly throughout the day if you want to lose weight.

The best analogy I can use to explain this is that you want to keep your metabolism firing throughout the day, so think of it as a camp fire, where you are consistently throwing small twigs or branches onto the fire to keep it going rather than throwing two or three large logs on it at once.

Think of how you feel after eating a massive meal. You are probably bloated, tired and without a lot of energy. This is because your body is working overtime to process and deal with all the food you have just consumed. Your body is also naturally geared to store a lot of this food as fat, which isn't going to help your weight-loss efforts.

On the other hand, eating small portions throughout the day gives your body enough time to process the food efficiently and keeps your metabolism firing. It will also aid in keeping your blood-sugar levels stable, as you are eating regularly.

I call these meals 1–5 (with an optional meal 6) and suggest eating every two to three hours throughout the day. If you are training regularly, you will also find that you are hungrier during the day, which is a great sign that you are on the right track and your body is in the best possible position to burn fat.

The other thing about cravings is that one can lead to the next and this can become a vicious cycle. It can be a hard cycle to break, and the first week can be especially tough, but once you have broken the cycle by eating foods that have a high nutritional value, you will find that your cravings will diminish or disappear entirely.

DITCH THE CALORIE COUNTING!

I know calorie counting is one of the most popular methods employed in weight-loss programs today, but I strongly encourage you to stop focusing on how many calories are in a particular recipe or how many you have consumed each day. Instead, I would like you to focus on the actual nutritional value of the food. For example, some calorie-counting diets will tell you that you can eat whatever you like, as long as you stay under a certain number of calories per day. With that logic you could choose to use up your calories eating ice-cream, a burger and a glass of wine, which could end up being the only foods you put into your body for a whole day. This is just crazy and totally lacks any focus on fuelling your body correctly! Does this make any sense to you? Do you think that this type of mentality promotes long-term, sustainable weight loss?

The other issue I have with calorie counting is that, for a busy woman, there just isn't enough time in the day. I know there are phone apps and calculators to help you track your intake, but I can't think of anything worse than having to constantly input and record what I'm eating. I believe you are better off focusing on eating foods that are good for you and will actively help you to lose weight. If you can learn to enjoy these types of foods and embrace my 80:20 rule, then you can finally kick calorie counting to the kerb once and for all!

This is the reason why you won't find a macro-nutrient breakdown or calorie count for any of the recipes in this book or on the 'Kim's Kitchen' section of my website. What you will find is a lot of tasty, simple and practical recipes that are suited to a busy family lifestyle and are all about real foods to help you stay healthy.

PAIRING YOUR MACROS CORRECTLY

I truly believe in embracing all food groups as part of a healthy lifestyle. When it comes to weight loss, it is important to pair the right macronutrients together at the right times of day to maximise results. ('Macronutrients' is a term to describe where your body gets its energy from. The three macronutrients that play essential roles in the body are carbohydrates, fats and proteins.) This is the approach I always take and it has helped thousands of women achieve their weight-loss goals and maintain the body shape they want.

Here is a breakdown of different foods, grouped according to what macro category they predominantly fit under and with some advice about pairing them throughout the day.

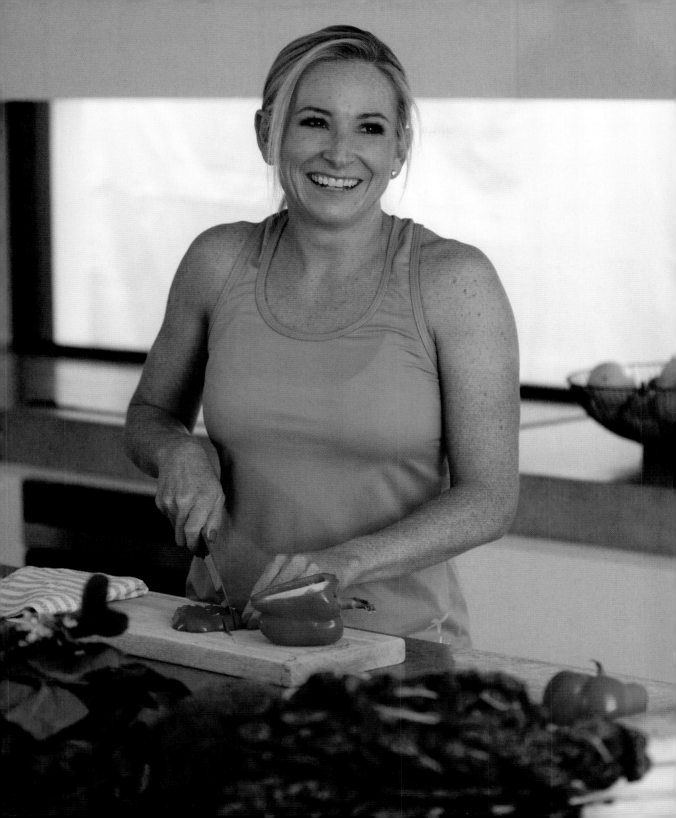

Carbohydrates

Good sources of carbohydrates are critical to provide the energy your body needs to train hard and get through the day. A good source of carbohydrate is high in fibre and low GI. Some examples of these are oats, brown rice, quinoa and sweet potato.

Highly processed carbohydrates that you need to steer clear of (especially if weight loss is your goal) are found in white bread, white rice and many common breakfast cereals, just to name a few. In refined foods like these, the carbohydrates have been stripped of their goodness and offer no real nutritional value. Later on in the book, I will share a full list of foods to embrace every day and some foods that I choose to stay away from and why.

Protein

Protein is simply amazing! Not only does it have a minimal effect on your blood sugar, it will also keep you fuller for longer and it is the real building block that our bodies rely on to stay strong and make repairs. Protein helps us build muscle and the more lean muscle that you have on your body, the more fat you will burn each and every day. If you are trying to lose weight then including a small amount of protein in every meal is the way to go!

Some examples of good sources of protein are chicken, pork, fish, eggs, tofu and cottage cheese. Some poorer choices of protein are foods such as deep-fried chicken or nuggets, or any highly processed meats, such as luncheon meat or salami.

Fats

Let's clear up a common misconception: that all fats make you fat. Actually, eating good fats will not make you fat; in fact, eating the right amount of good fats will help you lose weight. Good fats have the ability to keep you feeling fuller for longer, aid in keeping your blood-sugar levels stable and – best of all – they can actually help improve your mood. Some great examples of foods with good fats are salmon, nuts, seeds, olive oil and avocado.

When it comes to fats, it is really important to know the good from the bad. Think about where the foods come from. Good fats will generally occur naturally – think of avocados coming from a tree or salmon coming from the ocean – bad fats are most commonly processed, such as margarine or vegetable oil, which are highly processed. These will not help you lose weight and I don't believe they are beneficial for you in any way.

So, now I have explained all the benefits of the different macronutrients, here are some suggestions for pairing them correctly throughout the day to maximise weight loss.

Meals 1, 2 & 3 – Breakfast, morning tea and lunch
In these meals you are aiming to pair good sources of carbohydrates with a small amount of protein. The reason for this is that the good sources of carbohydrates give you energy in the earliest part of the day when you need it most. As I mentioned before, you want to include a small amount of protein in every meal to help keep you fuller for longer and also to assist in regulating your blood-sugar levels.

Meals 4, 5 & 6 – Afternoon tea, dinner and an optional evening snack
Later in the day, your body doesn't require as much energy, so you are aiming to pair good fats with protein as the basis for each meal. The great thing about protein and good fats is that they have a minimal effect on your blood-sugar levels and therefore they put your body into a fantastic fat-burning position.

If you stick to these principles and eat regularly throughout the day I promise that you will feel better, have more energy and lose weight. I also endorse these principles as a way of eating for general health. It's the way I eat every single day and although my goal is not weight loss it helps me maintain the weight and shape I want.

THE TRUTH ABOUT FOOD AND WEIGHT LOSS
For years, people have believed – and have been encouraged to believe – that the key to weight loss is dependent on how hard you train. I am here to tell you this is simply not true. Here is the truth:

WHAT YOU EAT WILL ACCOUNT FOR 80 PER CENT OF YOUR WEIGHT-LOSS RESULTS!

Your focus should be on what you eat, not how hard you train. Training is important, don't get me wrong, but there is no way that you can out-train a bad diet. I've lost track of the number of times I have heard people say, 'I have had a big weekend: I need to get back into the gym on Monday.' I totally understand the need and want to train, but the reality is that your results are really going to come from the thought and time you put into your meals and not the distance you do on the rowing machine.

If your current mindset is based around training to burn off poor food choices then this needs to change, as you will be constantly chasing something you will never achieve in a healthy, sustainable way. Once you accept that 80 per cent of your results will come down to what you eat, you will be on the right path to successful long-term weight loss.

'You can't out-train a bad diet.'

REAL FOODS THAT FUEL POSITIVE NUTRITION

By now you should understand my philosophy of Positive Nutrition (or 'real food') and the differences between eating healthily and eating for weight loss.

I want to give you a brief description of more than 50 foods that are highly beneficial for fuelling your body correctly. I also want to outline some foods that I choose to steer clear of and tell you why. This is not a complete list of what to eat and what not to eat, but it will provide you with some idea of the foods that I recommend and why some are more beneficial than others.

I have broken these down into the three different 'macro' categories: carbohydrates, proteins and fats. This should help you with pairing the right foods at the right time of day. Please keep in mind that, when I list a food under a certain heading, it's because it predominantly falls under that food category. All food tends to contain three core macros in some way, but I am thinking about the dominant macro in each food.

If you are not familiar with some of these ingredients, take the time to have a close look at the ever-expanding health-food section of your supermarket. All these foods are also readily available online or at your local health-food store. I just love the fact that these foods are now becoming commonly available and accessible in mainstream society.

GOOD SOURCES OF CARBOHYDRATES

Portion size for carbohydrates is no more than ½ cup (for grains, that is when cooked). Vegetable portion sizes are unlimited; and the greener the better.

Amaranth – Naturally gluten free, high in protein and it can be eaten as a seed or puffed.

Apple – A great source of fibre and antioxidants. Just make sure that you keep the skin on, as that is where the fibre is.

Asparagus – Easy to prepare, high in fibre and really quick to cook on the sandwich press.

Banana – High in potassium and fibre, and good for your digestion. Perfect to use on your oats.

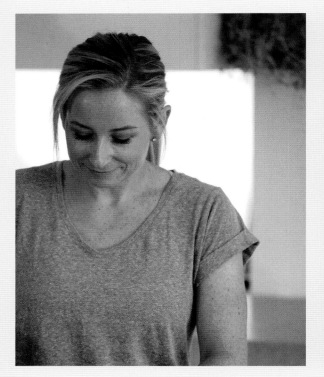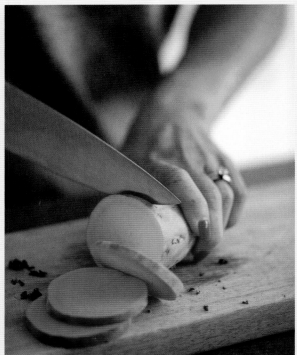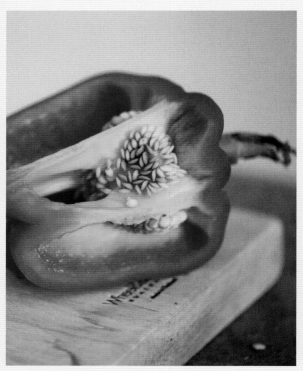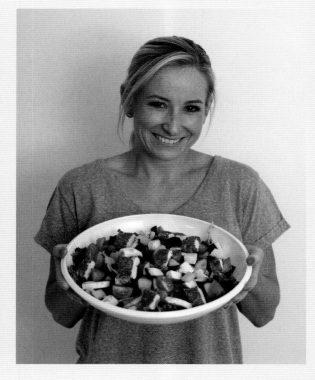

Berries – Nature's candy! High in antioxidants, they add natural sweetness to any dish. If weight loss is your goal and you love fruit, berries are your best go-to option.

Broccoli – Another green favourite, high in fibre and so easy to work into meals.

Brown rice – A great staple to have in your pantry and so much better for you than its white counterpart; it is low GI and high in fibre.

Capsicum – Adds bold flavour and a bit of colour to meals.

Carrot – Full of fibre and a great snack to take with you when you are on the go.

Cauliflower – You can do so much with it. I even make fried rice with it! Find my Cauliflower Fried Rice recipe on my website.

Celery – Full of vitamins and great to use with dips.

Couscous – A great carbohydrate option but be mindful to stick strictly to portion size.

Lemon – Aids digestion. I have lemon water every morning as a way to kickstart the day.

Lentils – A great source of carbohydrates and protein. A fabulous option for vegetarians.

Mushrooms – I eat mushrooms all the time. They fill you up and they are also a great source of iron.

Oats – I eat oats every day for breakfast (see recipe, page 129). They are high in fibre and provide a great source of energy to kickstart your day.

Onion – Adds flavour to any meal.

Pasta – There are so many great pastas available today, such as buckwheat, amaranth, rice or wholemeal. It is important to stick strictly to the correct portion size and not overeat.

Quinoa – This grain is very special. It isn't only a good carbohydrate, it is also high in protein and gluten free. This should be another staple in your house.

Rye bread – Bread should be limited if your goal is weight loss, but a couple of slices one or two times per week is fine. Rye bread is preferable, as it is higher in fibre then other breads.

Spinach – One of my favourite greens. It is packed full of nutrients and vitamins.

Sweet potato – I LOVE sweet potato! It is so easy to cook and extremely versatile. Lid down on the sandwich press for 30 seconds and you are good to go.

Teff – The world's smallest grain! It is high in protein, gluten free and extremely versatile. I use it in everything from soups (see page 153) to chicken nuggets (see page 152)

Zucchini – Really versatile and great as an alternative to noodles (if you have a spiraliser).

PROTEINS

Portion size for protein works by comparing it to the size of your palm, or around 100 grams per serve. Remember that protein has a minimal effect on your blood-sugar levels, so having a little more or a little less won't negatively affect your results.

Beef – Lean beef once or twice a week is a great source of iron.

Chicken – I would always suggest free-range or organic. It is a great and affordable protein source.

Eggs – Organic or free-range are best. A fantastic, wholesome combination of protein and fat.

Fish – High in omega-3 fatty acids and easy to digest.

Ham – Leg ham is good for a quick, tasty snack.

Pork – A great lean protein. I use it a lot in my recipes.

Tofu – The go-to protein source for vegetarians. Even for those who aren't vegetarian, it is really nice when marinated.

Turkey – A great alternative to chicken. You can either buy raw turkey breast, cook and slice, or buy precooked from the butcher or deli.

Cottage cheese – A great meat-free source of protein and extremely versatile.

Feta cheese – A small amount is great to add a bit of zing to your meals.

Milk – Having a small amount of milk each day is totally fine, whether it is full cream, low fat or a non-dairy alternative such as rice or almond milk. Just be mindful that if your goal is weight loss, then moderation is important.

Parmesan cheese – A great way to add a sharp flavour to any meal, especially in omelettes. Allow around 1 tablespoon per serve.

Yoghurt – look out for a good Greek-style yoghurt that's higher in protein and lower in sugar and fat. The sugar and fat content per 100 grams should be less than 5 grams.

FATS

Almonds – These are high in fats and protein, so it's essential that you stick to the portion size; maximum 15 per serve.

Chia seeds – A total superfood, high in protein and good fats. I mix it in with my oats every morning. There are too many benefits to live without this tiny seed.

Olive oil – Should be cooked on medium heat or less to retain its health benefits.

Peanut butter – Make sure there is only one ingredient in it; that it's 100 per cent peanuts.

Sesame seeds – Something you can throw easily into meals 4, 5 or 6.

MISCELLANEOUS

Chilli – A great way to fire up your metabolism and add some heat to your dishes.

Cinnamon – This is great at keeping your blood-sugar levels stable and also fantastic at adding a bit of sweetness to any meal.

Curry powder – Adds flavour and packs a punch.

Garlic – Strengthens your immune system and adds a delicious flavour.

Smoked paprika – Full of vitamins and great for adding flavour to savoury dishes.

Psyllium husks – A great way to add fibre to any meal.

Pure maple syrup – It's very important that you purchase maple syrup that has nothing added to it. It will be a bit more expensive, but totally worth it.

Rice cakes – These are great for most meals. They are so low in macros that they can easily be used as a staple for any meal. Add either carbohydrates and protein or good fats and protein on top.

Rice malt syrup – Less processed than standard white sugar. A small amount is a great way to add sweetness.

Tamari – This gluten-free version of soy sauce is a great marinade option that tastes amazing.

Yeast extract spread – Yeast extract spreads such as Vegemite, Marmite and AussieMite are extremely good mixed with cottage cheese.

DRINKS

Apple cider vinegar – Good for your digestive system. I add two teaspoons to my lemon water every morning when I get up.

Coffee – Have a maximum of two coffees per day, preferably black or with just a dash of milk.

Green tea – A delicious way to aid weight loss and reap its health benefits.

Kombucha – This aids gut health, but be mindful of the sugar content.

Peppermint tea – A great tea to have prior to bedtime, as it has no caffeine.

Water – Drink a minimum of two litres per day, breaking it down so you are consuming two small glasses after each meal throughout the day.

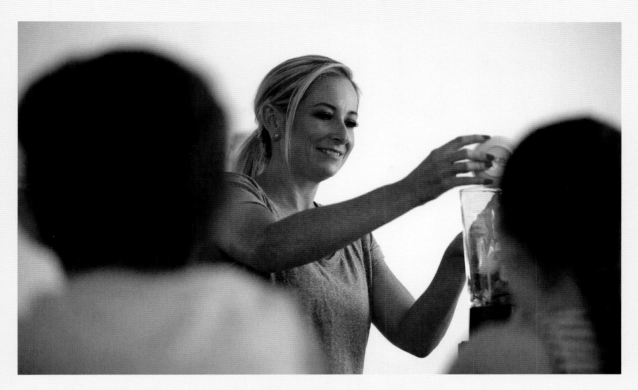

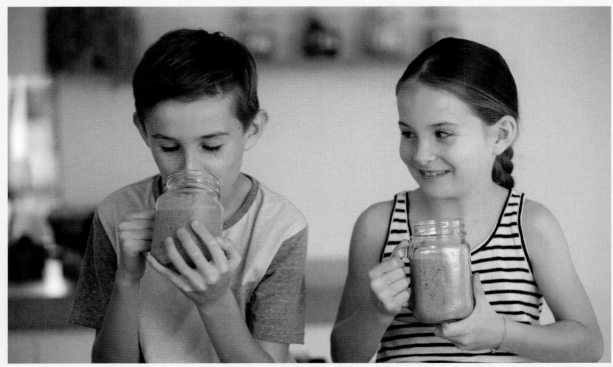

MY 'NO-GO' LIST!

Here are the foods that I choose to steer clear of or have only very occasionally.

Diet soft drinks – You don't need them: they provide zero nutritional value.

Soft drinks – Zero nutritional value and full of sugar, so avoid them at all costs.

Sports drinks – Designed for athletes to avoid dehydration and loss of electrolytes. High in sugar so they are best avoided.

Fruit juices – Look carefully at the sugar content as it is usually really high, especially in juice targeted at kids. If you do want to have juice, make it yourself or buy freshly squeezed – that way you can include vegetables such as carrot or kale that are lower in sugar.

Fried foods – Anything deep-fried is not going to be beneficial for you. There are better ways to cook food.

Chocolate – A combination of sugar and fat, which is what you want to avoid if weight loss is your goal. If you are going to have chocolate, choose one with a 70 per cent or higher cacao content. And limit yourself to a small piece.

Lollies – Highly processed simple sugars will spike your blood-sugar levels.

White bread – Highly processed and usually includes added sugar. There are so many better alternatives.

Margarine – Stick with butter, it is a far better choice.

White rice – Has been stripped of all its goodness. Brown rice is all you need!

Processed meats – Do yourself a favour by focusing on lean cuts of meat instead.

White flour – Has been bleached and processed. There are so many flours available today that will work just as well; for example, buckwheat, spelt and wholemeal.

Cakes – Keep them to birthdays only, when you can really enjoy a slice.

Ice-cream – This common go-to snack after dinner is not a great combination of sugar and fats. Check out my ice-cream recipe on page 186.

Frozen meals – I understand these are convenient, but fresh is always best.

Alcohol – Keep it to a minimum, especially if weight loss is your goal.

Alcohol

Let me say straight away that alcohol and weight-loss goals DO NOT MIX! Once you have achieved or are close to your goal then it is fine have a few drinks in moderation, but if you seriously want to lose weight, stay away from the alcohol.

To put it simply, the reason for this is that when there is alcohol in your system it is very hard, if not impossible, for your body to burn fat. So imagine for a moment that you are having one or two glasses of wine per night. Over the course of a week your body is never going to be in a true fat-burning position, regardless of how well you have eaten.

If your goal is to maintain a healthier lifestyle, then please remember the 80:20 rule when it comes to alcohol and drink in moderation. This is something I get asked about ALL the time, especially which drinks are better than others. This is a really difficult question to answer because ideally it is none, but in need of a response I normally suggest red wine or clear alcohol such as vodka served on the rocks or with soda water as the best options.

Please recognise there are also certain times in your life when you just need to totally relax and enjoy a few cocktails. It is at these times that you should focus on the moment, where you are and the people you are with rather than overthinking your nutrition. For me this happens only once or twice a year when I have escaped on holiday and am kicking back by a pool somewhere warm, enjoying the sunshine and time with my family.

The general rule of thumb for alcohol is to enjoy it in moderation, but if you feel you might have an issue in this area please talk to your doctor or a trusted friend, as having a healthy relationship with alcohol is an important part of a balanced lifestyle.

TAKEAWAY AND EATING OUT

I love to eat out and choose to enjoy it as part of my 80:20 balance. With that in mind, there are some options I choose ahead of others when it comes to different styles of takeaway food. Here is a very general guide to what to look for and what to avoid when it comes to eating out or having takeaway with family and friends.

TAKEAWAY OPTIONS

Burgers

I am not a huge burger lover but I am impressed with all the boutique burger places that have opened up, focusing on quality ingredients. I would personally choose one of these outlets ahead of the larger chain-style stores. Lean meat or chicken burgers are the best option, but go easy on the condiments and choose water and sweet potato fries to go with your meal.

Fish and chips

Most places will provide a grilled fish option and that should always be the go-to over beer battered and deep-fried. Opt for a salad rather than chips and, again, go easy on the sauces.

Pizza

For me pizza tends to fall into two categories: low-price mass-produced pizza and gourmet pizza made with high-quality produce. I would never buy pizza based on the price alone and would always choose the high-quality option.

Chicken

Steer clear of fried options and choose grilled. You should have lots of salad choices available and this can easily be made into a healthy meal.

Subs & sandwiches

Most sandwich counters now have flatbread or wraps available rather than sugary white breads. If you stay away from highly processed meats, this can be a very healthy option.

When you're hungry your body is craving nutrients.

Choose the right fuel.

EATING OUT

What I love about eating out these days is that you can always ask for modifications to the menu to get exactly what you want. This is especially important if you are on a journey to lose weight, in which case I would strongly advise checking out the restaurant's menu before you arrive so you are clear on what you are able to order.

Asian cuisine

Asian food can sometimes be tricky as there are lots of sauces and marinades used. Try to stick to plain options like steamed vegetables and fish.

Mexican

I think Mexican is a great option for a healthy meal out. Don't be afraid to tell them exactly what you want; for example, I always make sure to ask for brown rice and guacamole while holding the cheese and sour cream.

Sushi

I love sushi as it is usually made fresh to order. Substitute white rice for brown rice and stay away from anything deep-fried.

Italian

When you think about the sauces, pasta choices can be difficult, but there are some wonderful Italian meal options with lean meats, chicken, fish and vegetables. So, rather than ordering the pasta, stick to the 'real food' options.

Indian

Indian cuisine is difficult, as everything seems to be based around white rice, naan bread and heavy sauces. Keep in mind portion size and focus on dishes without cream, such as tandoori chicken.

Spanish/Greek/Middle Eastern

You should have some really great meal options here, with lean meats and fantastic salads full of flavour. It's one of the best options when it comes to dining out at a restaurant.

NUTRITION AND TRAVELLING

When you travel regularly, I know how difficult it can be to choose healthy eating options, especially if you are trying to lose weight. I am a little bit more relaxed about this these days than I used to be, after a rather embarrassing incident at Nadi Airport in 2014. I was singled out by Fijian customs for trying to import what they thought was a commercial quantity of tuna!

My advice, when it comes to short flights that only last a couple of hours or fewer, is to steer clear of airline food all together and simply eat before you fly. On longer flights where you need to eat, take some snacks with you, such as almonds or homemade protein balls (see my recipe on page 185) and preselect a meal that suits you on the plane. In my experience, the gluten-free option is often a good healthy choice.

In hotels, don't be scared to ask for exactly what you want and be very careful with the breakfast buffet, as portion size can easily go out the window. I find that if I train early in the morning when I am travelling, even if it is just a walk, I am more likely to make better food choices at breakfast, which then sets me up to make better choices throughout the day.

'Gym work is great but real transformation happens when you consistently change what you put into your mouth every day.'

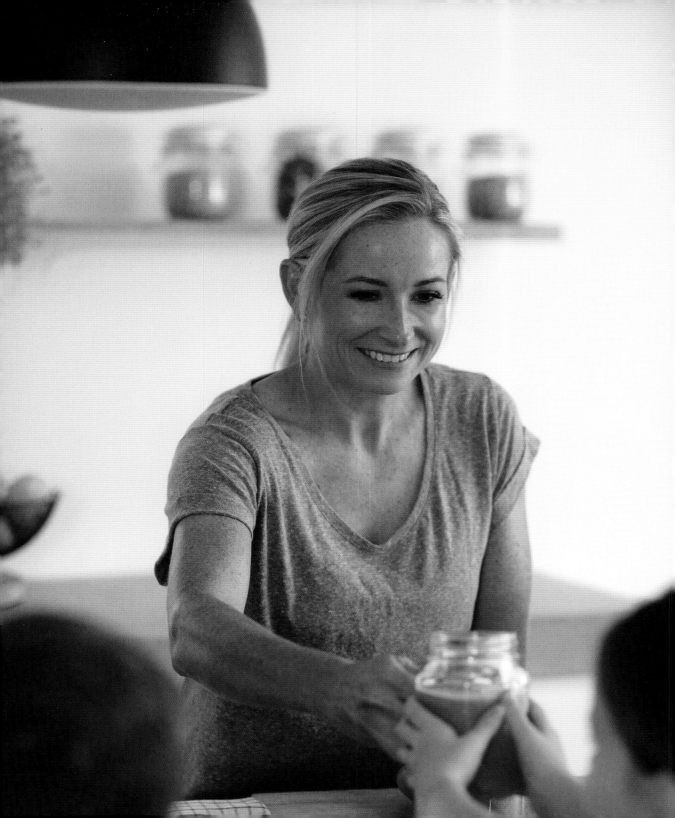

SUPPLEMENTS

I get asked a lot about nutritional supplements and I always answer that a normal, healthy person should be getting the nutrients they need if they are eating good foods regularly. Having said this, you might require supplements for health reasons, or wish to add them into the mix if you are doing serious training or have a specific need.

Here are some common supplements and my thoughts on each of them.

- BCAAs (Branched-chain amino acids) – If you are training heavily with weights these will assist in your recovery and can be sipped during your workout. Once again, they are for serious weight training only.
- Chlorophyll – Add to water to benefit your overall health.
- Multivitamins – Great for people who are not eating the right balance of foods each day.
- Olive oil extract – One hundred per cent natural and assists in regulating your blood pressure.
- Probiotic – Gut health is important when it comes to your overall wellbeing. A quality probiotic is part of my morning ritual and aids digestion.
- Protein powder – Find one that is low in sugar. Remember, it is not a meal replacement and should be taken after weight-training sessions only.

ANNA'S STORY

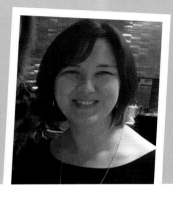

I wanted to say a massive thanks to you and the team for helping me to lose 19 kilograms so far, and teaching me how to look after myself so I'll never again have to 'start a diet'.

I contacted Kim after I weighed in at my heaviest weight ever, with my BMI at 30. The tipping point was going shopping and buying the next size up, again, and I realised something had to change.

I knew all the reasons (and excuses) why I had put on the weight, but just couldn't find a way to lose more than a few kilos before derailing, and each time putting on a bit more weight. I decided enough was enough and committed myself to Kim's program after seeing a friend's success.

As usual, I prepped my partner that I was starting yet another healthy eating plan and his response was, 'But you're always so cranky when you diet!' Believe me when I say he was right, but that is all in the past. I can honestly say I've not been 'cranky diet girl' for one second, as Kim's approach is not a diet, it is learning a new way of eating, and learning to develop a healthy relationship with food.

I was so happy with my nine-kilogram loss in the first eight weeks, and then another seven kilograms in the next eight weeks. I have just completed my third round, losing a total of twenty kilograms so far.

For the first time in a very long time I have a healthy relationship with food, and am so happy to have found an easy way of looking after myself again.

Anna

LESLEY'S STORY

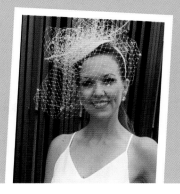

I'm your average 38-year-old mother of three living on the beautiful Gold Coast. Although my weight was considered healthy as far as national standards, I was never quite satisfied that this was it for me.

On starting Kim's program I, like most ladies, questioned whether I could stick to it and commit to the exercise component, but I just jumped right in and off I went. I found that the eating plan suited me and I also chose eight weeks in the year when there wasn't much happening in my calendar, so as to not be tempted to make poor choices. Although I was tempted on occasion, I made great choices and it had no effect on my results.

I am not going to lie; the first week was like having a hangover that didn't go. This just proved how much non-nutritious food I was feeding my body. But after the headaches were over I felt fabulous. I found that the further I went into the program, the more determined I was to get amazing results. My body changed in ways I never thought possible. My skin was clean and clear, I was never bloated, I was gaining definition all over my body and I caught myself second-glancing in the mirror, because I wanted to be certain that what I was seeing was right (abs and guns)!

Along the way, I got amazing support from Anni, Geraldine, Kim and most significantly the inspirational women who were smashing it out with me. No question was too silly. Without this support, I'm not sure I would have stuck it out.

I'm a few months post-program now and I still live by Kim's principles. I have not gained any weight and I know that, should I lose it for a while, I can come back and do it again. It's amazing what this process can do for your confidence. I am completely hooked on the Kim Beach philosophies.

Lesley

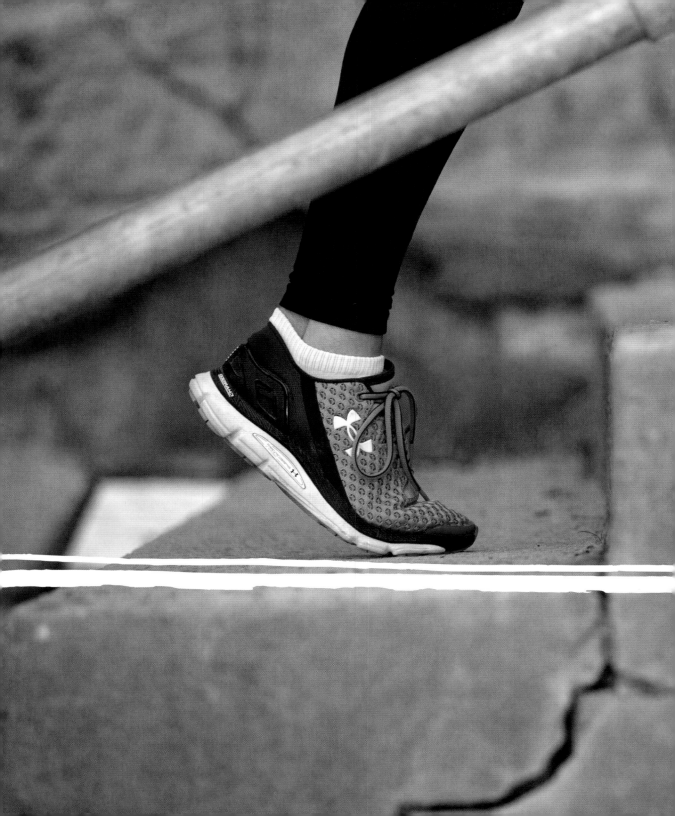

THE IMPORTANCE OF TRAINING

Chapter 4

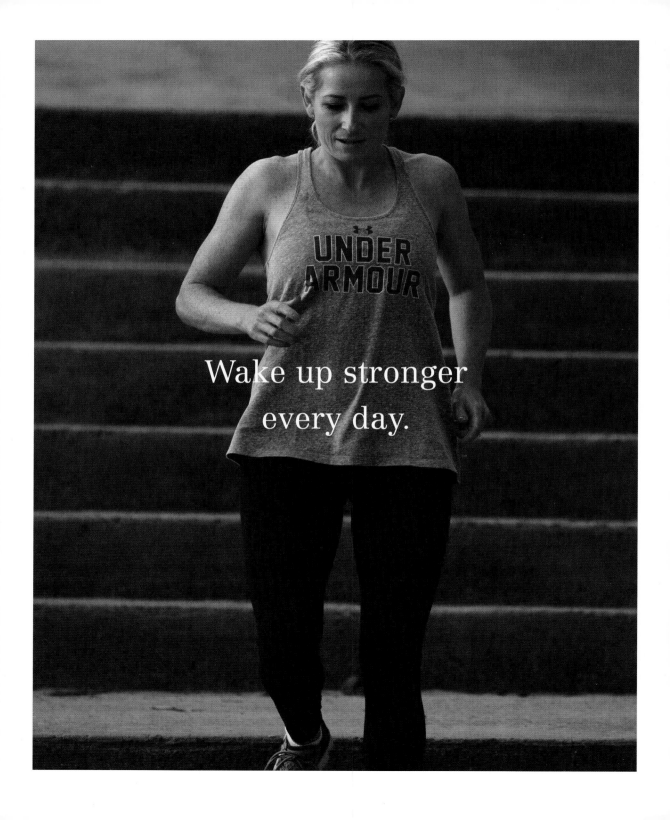

Wake up stronger
every day.

By now you'll have realised the importance of nutrition when it comes to your health and fitness. I also want you to know that training and exercise is a critical part of the mix, but is often an area that can be confusing and misunderstood. My objective in this section is to lay out all the different training options and help you to understand which ones to incorporate into your own personal regime to ensure you achieve your goals.

I really believe that it is called 'training' for a reason, as you are working towards something bigger. Training should have a purpose and you should definitely set goals around what you are trying to achieve. If you don't do this, training can easily become boring and the excuses will start to kick in.

Regular training has SO many health benefits for your body and mind. Whether it is to simply improve your fitness, so you have more energy to play with your kids, or you want to complete a triathlon, or if weight loss is a priority for you, training regularly is going to help you achieve your goal.

One of the key benefits to training — and one that is often downplayed — is the way it makes you feel good. Sure, you might not feel fantastic 35 minutes into a 40-minute spin class, but I guarantee that an hour after the class has finished you will be feeling on top of the world. The reason for this is that when you train, your body produces 'feel-good' hormones called endorphins.

Once you get into a regular training routine, you will very quickly see how this will positively affect your mood, mental sharpness and clarity. You will also find that this translates into having a lot more energy, and things like getting out of bed every morning and sleeping well throughout the night aren't just a dream anymore, they are a part of everyday life!

Your body is designed to move and it doesn't take kindly to long periods of inactivity or being treated badly. This is when you put on weight and health problems can occur. The best way to avoid this is to make friends with your body and train it regularly a few times per week. My favourite quote on this subject is: 'Treat your body as though it belongs to someone you love.' This is a mantra that I try to consider every single day.

There is no single routine that suits everyone and every goal, so it is really important to train according to what you are trying to achieve; for example, if your goal is to run a half marathon, then your training would be mostly made up of running. This may seem quite obvious, but what if your goal is weight loss or what if your goal is to shred (meaning to get you as lean as possible) and build muscle? They would both require completely different approaches to training than going on a long-distance run three to four times per week. It is the same if you have some limitations when it comes to physical activity: just set a goal and focus on the best way to achieve it.

A common mistake with training comes from those who adopt the popular all-or-nothing mentality. This means you will go from long periods of inactivity to training seven days per week at high intensity. This might provide some quick results but it is also hard on your body, which can lead to injury and exhaustion, and will work against you in the long term. Your training schedule needs to be something that is sustainable and fits into your normal life.

Choosing the right time to train and planning in advance are the two key factors when it comes to getting your training sessions done each week. So, if you know you are going out for dinner late on a Friday night, it probably isn't the smartest idea to book a 6am boxing class on Saturday morning, as you will inevitably end up skipping the class and feeling bad for having done so. Instead you could plan an 11am yoga class or an early afternoon walk with a friend, because they are both achievable and will fit properly into your schedule.

I find that Sunday is the best time for me to sit down and plan for the week ahead, and that goes for both my training and nutrition. I lock my training sessions into my calendar as I would any other meeting and this ensures that I set aside the time and make them a priority. There is honestly a real power that comes from writing things down: it makes everything clearer and is beneficial for those of us who are visual people. Saying that you are going to get up at 5am on Wednesday to do a spin class is very different from writing it in your diary and mentally committing to it ahead of time. Another great way to make sure you commit to your training sessions is to do a few each week with a friend. That feeling of letting someone else down can often be the difference between pulling yourself out of bed on a cold winter's morning, or rolling over and hitting the snooze button.

So let's look at how to set up your training week, depending on your goals.

'The more lean muscle you build on your body, the more fat you will burn at rest.'

GOAL 1: GETTING YOUR BODY MOVING – START TO TRAIN!

If you haven't exercised for a while, then you want to make sure you ease yourself into regular training. Depending on your level of fitness, I would recommend three or four half-hour walks per week. Find your rhythm with this for a few weeks and then start to increase the length and intensity of your walks. Set small goals each week and take the time when you are walking to think about your health, fitness and your new big, crazy goal.

GOAL 2: WEIGHT LOSS

So you have a reasonable level of fitness and you may have been trying to lose weight for a while. Your nutrition is now on point and it is time to match the training program to your weight-loss goal. For this, I would suggest three or four cardio sessions per week. Depending on your level of fitness, these could be a mix of light, moderate and high intensity sessions. You will want to include two full-body weight-training sessions each week. Please do not be scared of these, as I will explain all the wonderful benefits of weight training in the next section of the book. The weight sessions can be done in your own home or at the gym, based on what you are comfortable with.

GOAL 3: BUILD MUSCLE AND SHRED

This is a common goal for a lot of women who are within a few kilos of their ideal weight but want to improve their shape and build muscle. This goal requires a heavy focus on weight training three or four times per week and a couple of high-intensity cardio workouts.

You can see from the above suggestions that different goals require very different approaches to training and it is important to build a training regime that fits your goals and suits your lifestyle. A great option, if you are unsure about how to approach this, is to book time with a qualified personal trainer at your local gym, so you can sit down, discuss and create a personalised training plan. Or visit www.kimbeach.com for more options.

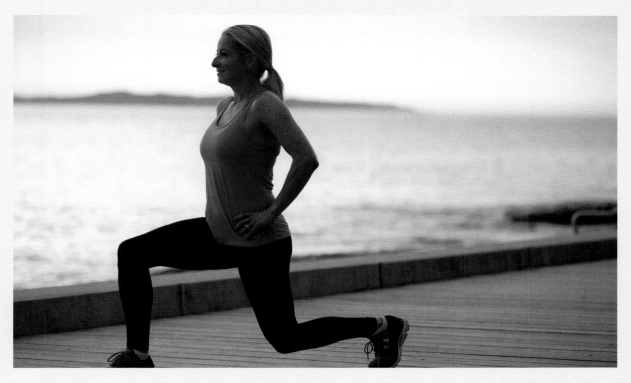

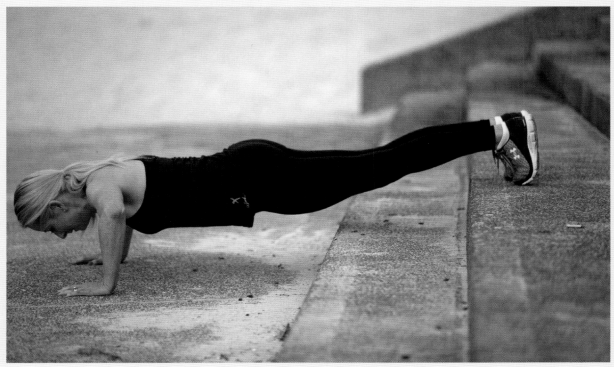

You will notice in each of the examples above that there are between one and three days of rest per week. Rest is as critical to the success of your routine as training and it should be planned for, just like any other training session. Your body and mind both need time to recover and this will enable them to come back stronger and sharper as time goes on. There may also be times when you need to take a complete break from your training and my advice is to listen to your body. If mental or physical fatigue is setting in, take a week off, get plenty of rest and be kind to your body. It is often after these weeks that you will find yourself completely re-energised and setting new personal bests.

Sometimes, it doesn't matter how well you have planned out your weekly schedule, life is going to throw some curve balls at you and your training week will be thrown into chaos. This is totally okay and normal, but please don't let one week translate into two or three unplanned weeks of chaos, as this is when you will find that your training will totally go off the rails. If you do have a few days where things are not going according to plan, then try and ramp up your incidental exercise each day. Maybe you could take the stairs instead of the lift, catch public transport and then walk to work rather than driving the whole way, or simply get outside and enjoy an impromptu game of football or soccer with your kids.

Don't forget that, aside from walking, running and training or attending classes at the gym, there are some amazing alternatives available that may better suit your pace. Exercise such as Pilates, spin classes, yoga, tai chi, skiing, rollerskating, horseriding, cycling, swimming, soccer, netball, touch football, triathlon, adventure racing, hockey, aquarobics, boot camps – the list is endless!

These activities all represent fantastic ways to get your body moving and can easily be incorporated into your training week, whatever your goals. Throwing a bit of variety into the mix is a great way to make sure you are enjoying your training and not getting bored with the same routine. Think about this: you can get the same workout from a game of touch footy as you can from a five-kilometre run, but the game of touch footy will probably be a lot more fun and time will fly by, because you are enjoying it with friends.

WHY EVERY WOMAN SHOULD TRAIN WITH WEIGHTS

When it comes to talking about training, this is my absolute favourite subject. If I could be granted one wish, it would be that every woman in the world would know and understand the phenomenal benefits of weight training.

Weight training, or resistance training, is simply lifting weights with the goal to build strength, increase muscle mass and reduce body fat. Sounds easy, right?

Unfortunately, many women will opt for cardio training instead of weight training. I speak to a lot of people about this subject and their apprehension over weight training seems to fall under one of these three reasons:

1. They are scared that they will build too much muscle and get bulky.

2. They are intimidated by the weights area at their gym.

3. They don't belong to a gym and have no idea of how they are able to do weight training at home.

I would like to deal with these one by one, to reassure you that weight training needs to become part of your training regime (if it isn't already) and share all the wonderful benefits that this type of training will bring into your life.

Let's deal with the first reason: that if you train with weights you will get bulky and look like a man. Unless your body is somehow producing an unnatural level of testosterone, it is impossible for you to bulk up in the same way as men do after consistent weight training over a period of time.

As females, our bodies simply do not produce enough testosterone to make this happen. What will happen is that, with the correct program, your body shape will start to transform. You will have more definition in your arms, shoulders, legs, butt and tummy. I promise you that you will not end up looking bulky or like a body builder. From personal experience, I know what it takes to get your body into that kind of shape and this is not going to happen with weight training a

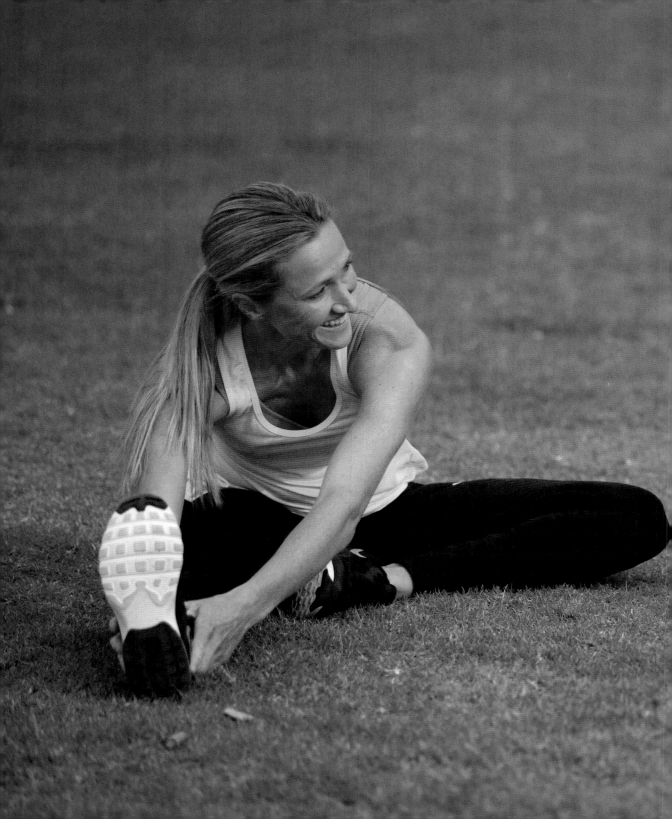

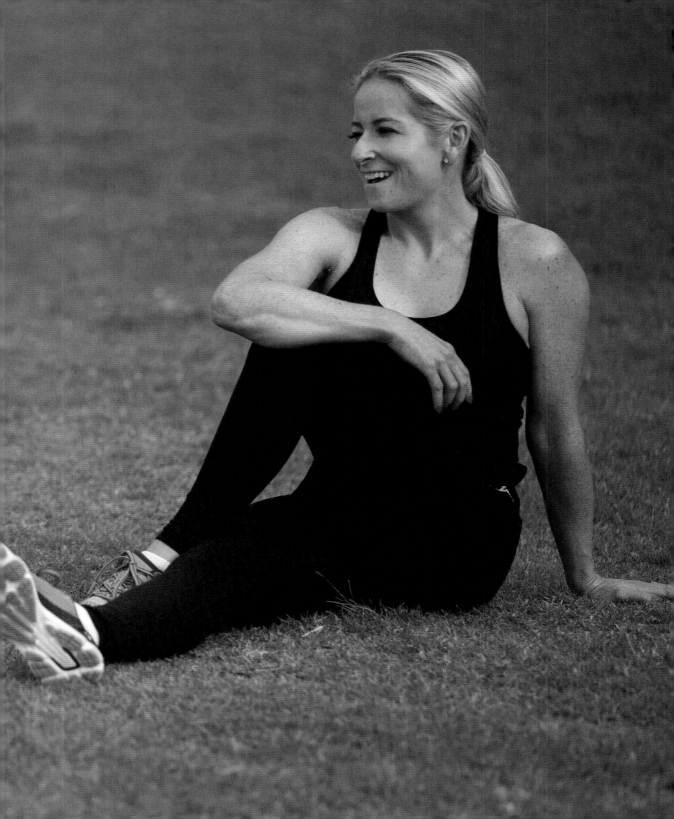

few days a week. You will notice, after a while, that your muscles will 'pop' during training, which is commonly called a 'pump'. This is just your blood rushing to your muscles and it is perfectly normal and actually good for you.

Secondly, let's discuss the fear that some women have of the weights area in their gym. I think that every woman who has ever visited a gym has encountered the moment when she looked over at the weights section of the gym and noted to herself that it was a male-dominated area filled with guys who easily throw weights around. Well, this might have been the case ten years ago, but now my gym is full of women focusing on weight training, which makes me very happy!

If you are apprehensive about entering the weights room, just pick a time of day when you know that it is going to be quiet to do your first few weights sessions, or, even better, book a couple of sessions with a personal trainer, who can create a proper program for you before walking you through the equipment that you will be using and showing you the correct techniques. There is no reason at all to be scared of the weights area and, once you have a couple of sessions under your belt, you will find that you belong there just as everyone else does.

The third common problem is that people don't belong to a gym and have no idea how to start weight training at home, which is totally understandable. As I see it, you have two clear options here: you either join your local gym (most will offer a free consultation and set up a program for you), or you buy some equipment and do your weights workouts at home. In the second scenario, all you need are some basic dumbbells, barbells and a program to follow. I know this is a popular option for mothers of young children or time-poor women in general, as it allows them to get their workout done early in the morning or in the evening without leaving home.

I hope this quashes some of the reasons that may have caused you to be apprehensive about adding weights into your training mix. If these explanations don't sway you, then check out all the other benefits that you are missing out on by not taking on weight training.

Regular weight training is going to make you physically stronger, which will result in you being more productive each day. Basic tasks, from working to playing with your kids, will be easier and you will have more energy to bring to them each day.

You will also become stronger on the inside, as your bone density will increase with consistent weight training. As you get older, your bone density decreases at a more rapid rate if you are not staying active, and lifting weights is an excellent way to fight this.

Another huge benefit of regular weight training is the shape you will develop and achieve over time. It's the only way to truly transform the shape of your body. If you have ever looked at the fitness models you see in magazines and online and wondered how they achieve their amazing physiques, I can assure you that they look the way they do with thanks to regular heavy weight training, rather than only doing cardio and gym classes.

Another way to think about this is the comparison between an Olympic sprinter and an Olympic marathon runner. They are both extreme examples, but each is built to perform a different task.

Lastly, I'm going to share with you the big secret of weight training: training regularly with weights will help you burn more fat 24 hours a day! The reason for this is that when you train with weights you build more lean muscle mass. Your body has to work very hard to maintain this muscle, which means you are constantly using more energy, even when you are at rest (for example, watching TV).

I control my weight through regular weight training. I absolutely love the shape it gives me and the way it makes me feel, so, if I haven't already convinced you, I want to stress again: I'm a HUGE fan of weight training and I think you should be too!

THE BENEFITS OF CARDIO TRAINING

There is no substitute for being physically fit and cardio is the only type of training that will help you achieve this. A solid training regime will include a mix of different types of cardio, as each one will offer you different benefits.

In technical terms, you measure the intensity of cardio by the number of heartbeats per minute. At one end of the scale, you have your resting heart rate and at the other end of the scale you have your maximum heart rate, which is 220 minus your age (e.g. if you are 40 years old your

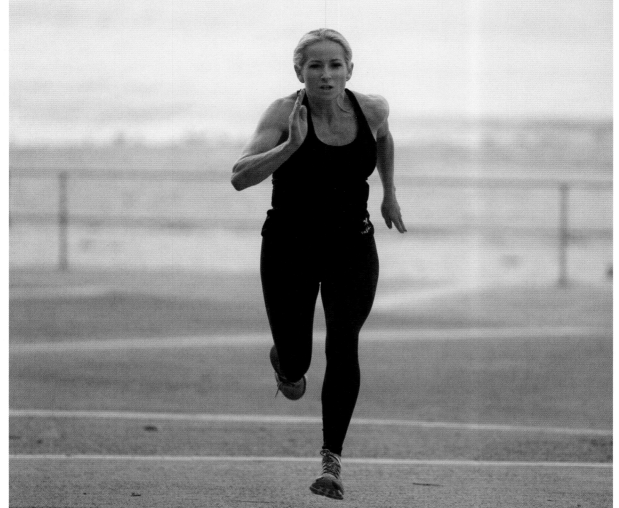

Train with passion
and intensity.

maximum heart rate should be 180 beats per minute). Much like calorie counting, I don't like to get fixated on this, so I would rather split cardio into three different areas – light, moderate and intense. Light cardio for me is when you can continue a conversation with a friend during a session. At the other end of the scale is intense cardio, where you are struggling to breathe, let alone have a conversation with anyone!

So, first let's look at light cardio. Light cardio sessions are a great idea if you are just starting your fitness journey. It is all about getting out and getting your body moving on a regular basis. They can also be great for a recovery session, or if you are getting back into your training after injury.

Some examples of light cardio sessions are:

- Walking
- Swimming
- Cycling

Basically, a light cardio session can last up to an hour and at no stage should you be out of breath.

Moderate cardio sessions are where you are getting your heart rate up to a certain point, but you are still able to have a 'puffy' conversation with a friend. These sessions are great for fat burning and are also fantastic at building your endurance and, of course, your level of fitness. If weight loss is your goal, I would recommend two of these moderate sessions per week, each between 45 and 60 minutes. Some examples of great moderate cardio sessions are:

- Power walk
- Run or jog
- Spin class or RPM class

Please keep in mind that everyone's fitness level is different, so some of the examples listed above might be intense sessions for you right now.

Moderate cardio sessions are great for burning additional fat while you are actually exercising, so the length of time is important. If you can build up to an hour over time, even if it's a power walk, this is going to be great for you and very important for weight loss.

HIGH INTENSITY INTERVAL TRAINING (HIIT)

I have a love–hate relationship with HIIT sessions. On the one hand, I love them as they can be done and dusted within 20 minutes, but on the other hand, they are really tough and can push your body to its limits. Please know that this type of training is hard and it can take some time to build your fitness to a level where you can complete it properly (please use your common sense).

HIIT sessions are designed to elevate your heart rate to a higher level with short periods of rest. This is why they are only usually around 20 minutes long; and by the end of it you should be toast! Another benefit of HIIT training is the positive impact it can have on your fitness level, considering the shortness of the sessions. Even long-distance athletes utilise HIIT as a key part of their training strategy.

Fat burning is another huge benefit of HIIT training. Your heart rate will stay elevated for hours after you have finished your training session, which means your body will continue to burn fat at a higher rate. Some examples of HIIT sessions are:

- Sprints
- Skipping
- Boxing

For a normal training regime, especially if weight loss is your goal, I would recommend two of these sessions every week.

EATING AND TRAINING

One question I am asked regularly is in relation to eating around your training sessions.

If weight loss isn't important to you, then the timing of eating your meals around training doesn't really matter, although I wouldn't suggest training on a full stomach.

If weight loss is your goal, then I would suggest that you eat a meal and then wait at least an hour before a cardio session or, even better, train on an empty stomach in the morning. For my morning sessions, I like to have a strong black coffee and then rip straight into my training. Always try to wait 30 minutes before you eat after your session, to maximise your fat-burning potential.

With weight training I suggest you eat before your session, as this will give you the energy you need to lift heavy weights. If you choose to incorporate a protein shake with your weight training have this straight after your session and remember it is not a meal replacement, so continue to eat as normal for the rest of the day.

'Always bring your A game.'

TAHNY'S STORY

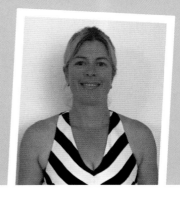

I have always had an interest in health and fitness but at times I have let other things get in my way. About three years ago my marriage came to an end and I found myself as a single mother with two children. Although I knew this was the best move forward for me, it was a difficult and challenging time that saw me gain about ten kilograms. It also meant that I had to work more days and getting to the gym was difficult. It was after a holiday in July last year that I realised it was time to get my weight and fitness back under control.

I started Kim's program August 2015 and decided that a big part of my success was going to be based on giving up alcohol. My tricky life had meant that I had been drinking regularly and the excess calories and sluggishness was not helping me in my hectic life.

Kim's approach to diet helped to regulate my blood-sugar levels and I went almost the full eight weeks with no alcohol. A major bonus was that I could do all the exercises at home with minimal equipment!

When I finished the program I just didn't want to stop: the fire to train hard had been relit and I needed to move forward. I decided to step it up a level. This meant pushing myself hard through the festive season and a family wedding, but I wanted to keep moving forward. I bought equipment to create a home gym in my carport and started training regularly.

Today I'm ten kilograms down and feeling amazing and full of energy. Exercise and healthy eating are definitely a part of my daily life now. I'm more positive and energised for the children I work with and my gorgeous and supportive family.

My goals for the future are to remain healthy and to put myself first so that I can be the best I can be for the people who need me.

Big hugs!

Tahny

KERRY'S STORY

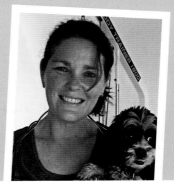

Back in 2004, I was 112.9 kilograms. I was a chef for 15 years and, in 2004, I returned home from living in the UK bigger than ever. I decided I needed a change so I worked my butt off and lost more than 30 kilograms with Weight Watchers. While I appreciate what that program did for me, looking back now, it really didn't teach me how to eat well. As long as you remain within your daily 30 points, you can eat what you like … and I often did!

When I started the #nolimits program I was sceptical as I had really struggled to lose anything in recent years. I thought I ate quite well generally, had been exercising six days a week for years and had even competed in four half-marathons … Why wasn't the weight shifting?

Then, eight weeks after I committed to living by Kim's advice, I felt like a new person. I lost a massive 7.2 kilograms and I wore a pair of skinny jeans to a hen's night, which felt AMAZING! My husband was smiling from ear to ear! I had so many compliments and all I could say was, 'KIM BEACH is AMAZING!' After once being a size 24, I am now a size 12!

I completing the program just before Christmas last year. It was tough, physically and mentally, but I made it through with results that I never expected. I was lifting heavy weights and starting to get definition. I was delighted. I won't lie, the process is tough but I truly believe that if I can do it, anyone can. Anyone can achieve things if they believe they can!

If someone asked me last year if I would be squatting 50 kilograms, only five kilograms from the slimmest I have been since school and would gain some AMAZING new friends, I would have laughed … but it's all true! This program has taught me so much about myself (physically and mentally), but most importantly confirmed that scales are not needed in my life.

Kerry

YOUR SEVEN-DAY PLANNER

Now that you understand what to eat and how to train in order to achieve your goals, I am going to help you put it all together in a simple weekly planner.

This planner is designed as a guide and it will show you how to structure a 'perfect' week, although (as we have discussed) a week is never perfect. So, if you do miss a meal or a training

	MONDAY	TUESDAY	WEDNESDAY
TRAINING	WEIGHTS – full body	HIIT – 10 x 40 metre sprints / 60 second recovery	MODERATE CARDIO – 500 metre swim 60% intensity
MEAL 1	Oats and Berries	Quinoa Brekky Bowl	French Toast
MEAL 2	Sweet Potato Devilled Eggs	Celery Boats	Turkey Wrap
MEAL 3	Chicken and Quinoa Meatloaf	Crunchy Turkey Salad	Tuna and Sweet Potato Patties
MEAL 4	Guacamole Crunch	Egg Burrito	Seed Bar
MEAL 5	Tamari and Maple Barramundi	Tandoori Chicken	Coconut Crumb Schnitzel
MEAL 6 / TREATS			Blueberry Chia Pudding

session, please don't write off the rest of the week, just pick yourself up and focus on the next day and remember it is all about consistency and not perfection!

Please feel free to change any of the meals during the week with another option with the same meal number. If you are looking for more information and options for meals and training, go to www.kimbeach.com.

THURSDAY	FRIDAY	SATURDAY	SUNDAY
WEIGHTS – full body	HIIT – Skipping 10 x 100 jumps / 60 second recovery	MODERATE CARDIO – 1 hour walk	REST
Oats and Berries	Brekky Smoothie	Choconana Pancakes	Big Breakfast Sausage
Carrot Cake Balls	Cinnamon Apples	Black Bean Dip with Vegie Sticks	Sweet Potato and Cauliflower Fritters
Sweet Mustard Chicken Salad	Asparagus and Quinoa Muffins	Chicken Nuggets	Creamy Broccoli Soup
Nori Wraps	Cucumber Boats	Five-minute Chocolate Cake	Turkey Cups
Pork San Choy Bau	Spicy Asian Prawns	Almond and Mint Encrusted Salmon	Chicken Satay Sticks
		Chocolate Gelato	

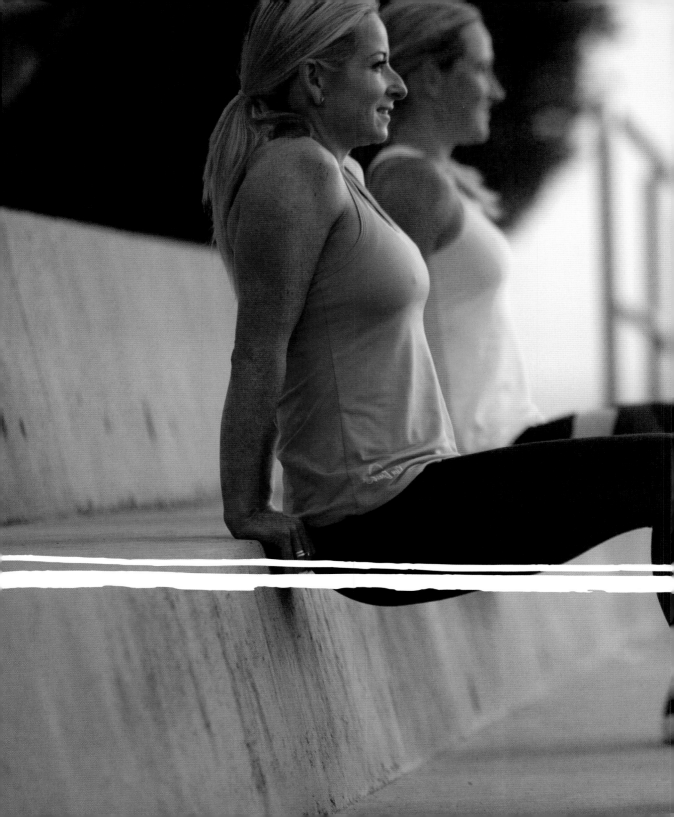

WEIGHT-TRAINING WORKOUTS

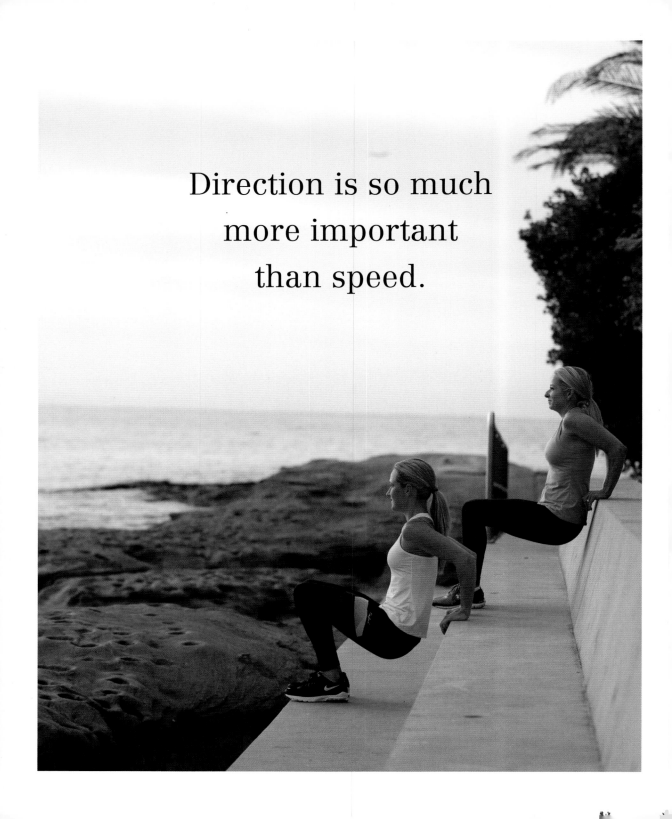

Chapter 5

Direction is so much more important than speed.

Here are two separate weight-training programs, both of which can be done from home using some dumbbells and an exercise ball. For your dumbbells, I recommend purchasing the adjustable type, so you can increase the weight as you become stronger over time.

The first weight-training program is a full-body workout that includes eight different exercises designed to work each major muscle group in your body. This workout is great for fat burning and is a fantastic entry-level program for you to begin your weights journey.

As you introduce yourself to the world of weight training, it's a good idea to stick to this weights workout twice a week for a four-week period. Record every session so you can see your progress along the way. Your aim should be to either increase the number of repetitions (reps) or weight for each exercise, each session. Then, after four weeks, it's time to change your training up so your body doesn't get used to doing the same thing.

Be mindful of the speed of every rep; for example, two seconds for the first phase of the movement and two seconds for the second phase. It's always preferable to take your time with each rep instead of just trying to get 15 reps out quickly. Focus on the muscles you are working and get the most out of every rep.

Towards the third set of every exercise, your muscles will start to experience fatigue, but keep going. If you can't get to 15 reps that's fine, but pump out as many as you can with perfect technique.

Record the number of reps you get out for each set, so you know what to try to improve on in your next session. This can also be a great motivator, especially four weeks down the track when you can see how well you've progressed.

It's really important that you warm up and cool down before and after any workout. This is a critical part of keeping your body at its peak, so you can give everything to your next session. A five-minute brisk walk before and after weight training is a great option.

The weights programs in this book are designed to target your whole body. To decide what is the right weight to start at for each exercise, you will need to spend your first weights session experimenting. Start off with a lighter weight and work your way up from there. Make sure you record each set you complete, including how many reps you manage to get out for each set and which weight you are using, so you have a measure to improve on in your next weights session. This is a great way to get competitive with yourself.

WEIGHTS PROGRAM #1

3 SETS X 15 REPS / 60 SECONDS REST BETWEEN EACH SET / SPEED 2:0:2*

Example: 15 x jumping squats, rest for 60 seconds, 15 x jumping squats, rest for 60 seconds, then 15 x jumping squats, rest for 60 seconds.

Refers to the speed of each repetition; for example, a push-up would be 2 seconds down, then 2 seconds up.

EXERCISES	DATE		DATE		DATE		DATE		DATE		DATE		DATE		DATE	
	REPS	WEIGHT	REPS	WEIGHT	REPS	WEIGHT	REPS	WEIGHT	REPS	WEIGHT	REPS	WEIGHT	REPS	WEIGHT	REPS	WEIGHT
Jumping Squats																
One-arm Row																
Push-ups																
Static Wall Squat																
Biceps Curl																
Triceps Kickbacks																
Mountain Climbers																
Lower Abs: Ins and Outs																

JUMPING SQUATS

This is a great exercise to start your session with: it will get your blood pumping and warm you up. Standing with feet shoulder-width apart and hands down by your side, bend down into a squat position, as if you are about to sit down in a chair, then jump up into the air using your arms to assist you and then straight back down into a squat again, so it becomes a continuous motion for 15 reps. This exercise will get your heart rate up so, after you have completed the 15 reps, use the whole 60 second recovery to prepare yourself for the next set. These will get easier the fitter you become, so stick with it!

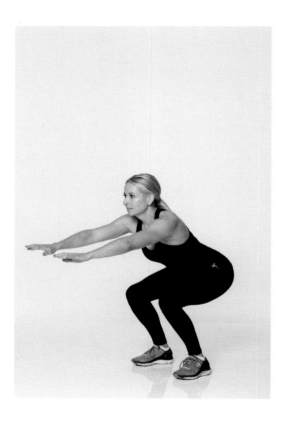
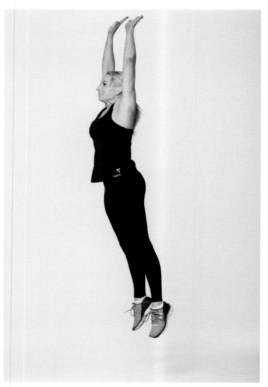

ONE-ARM ROW

You will need an exercise ball and a dumbbell for this exercise. If you have a training bench or a low table, feel free to use it instead of the exercise ball. Place one hand on the exercise ball, leaning your body forward so, for example, your right hand is on the exercise ball and your right knee is bent and supporting your weight. Keep your back flat and abdominals tight, while still breathing normally. With your left hand, hold the dumbbell straight down towards the floor and focus on bringing your elbow up to the sky, squeezing your shoulderblades together, then slowly lower the weight back down. Your hand should be in close to your rib cage and stay close to your body throughout the movement. Breathe out as your hand goes up to your rib cage, then breathe in as you lower the weight down to the starting position. Complete 15 reps then bring your body across to the opposite side of the exercise ball, swap hands and change leg position and complete 15 reps, rest for 60 seconds then repeat twice more.

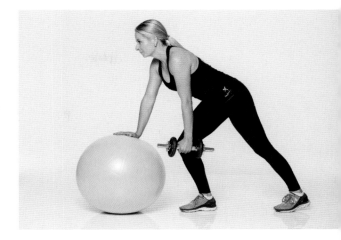

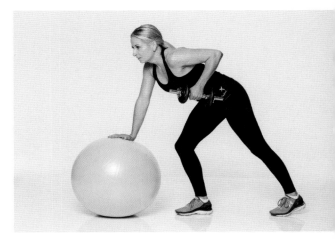

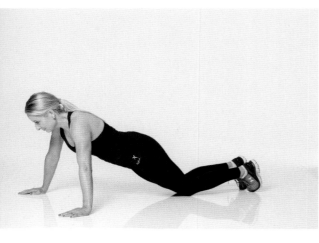

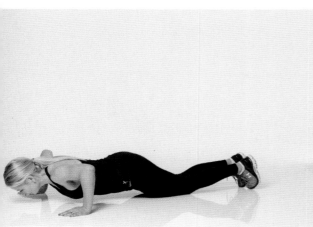

PUSH-UPS

You can do push-ups on your knees or on your toes, depending on where you're at with your strength. Start on your knees and make sure that at the finishing position on the downward phase, the angle at your elbow joint is at 90 degrees. Once you can do that for three sets of 15 reps, you can progress to push-ups on toes.

Push-ups on knees: Start with your hands slightly wider than shoulder-width apart and resting your body weight on your knees. Keep your back and bottom in line with each other and abdominals tight. If you feel any tension in your lower back, stop and refocus. Make sure your abdominals are tight and your lower back is not dipping forward or sticking out. The movement is coming from your elbow joint only, so your body should stay still and the muscles of your elbow joint need to step up and do the work. Bend at your elbow joint down to 90 degrees and then push up, without locking your elbow joint. Keep the speed controlled, working on two seconds down while breathing in and two seconds back up while breathing out.

Push-ups on your toes: Up on your toes, place your hands slightly wider than shoulder-width apart. Make sure your bottom is not dipping forward too far or sticking up. Bend at your elbow joint down to a nice 90-degree angle, then slowly come back up without locking your elbow joint. Breathe in on the way down and out on the way up. You may find that you can only get one set of push-ups on your toes out before you lose form, and that is fine. Complete one set on toes and then two sets on knees. This is a great exercise that will take time to perfect but, as they say, 'practice makes perfect'. Remember, it is not a race! If you can't get 15 out, record how many you managed to do and this will be the number you need to try to beat in your next session.

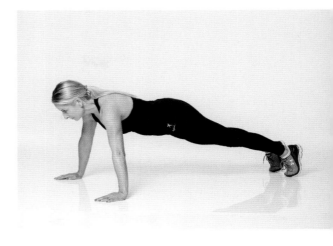

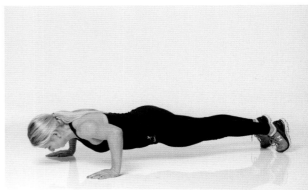

STATIC WALL SQUAT X 60 SECONDS

The static wall squat is a great leg burner and is also a fantastic exercise that can be done anywhere, with or without dumbbells. Find a wall, stand up against it and bring your feet forward. Slide down the wall until your knee joint reaches 90 degrees and hold that position for 60 seconds, while breathing normally. Then stand up, walk around and rest for 60 seconds. Repeat twice more for a total of 3 sets.

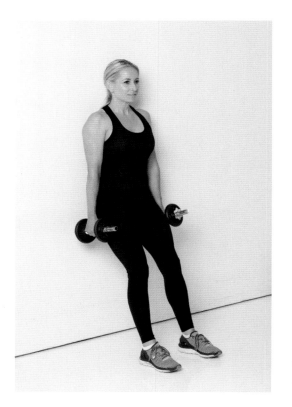
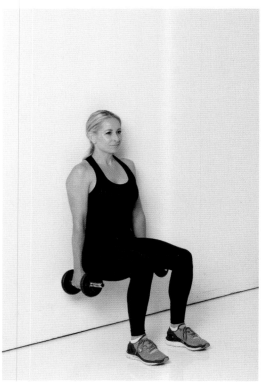

BICEPS CURLS

Stand with feet shoulder-width apart, knees slightly bent, holding a dumbbell in each hand down by your side. Bring the dumbbells up so your hands are in front of your shoulder joint and then extend slowly back down. It is very important that your body stays completely still throughout the movement and your abdominals are switched on. Breathe out as your arms are curling in and breathe in as your arms extend back down.

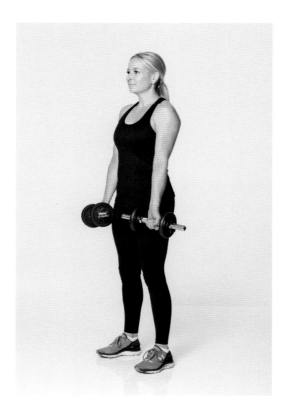
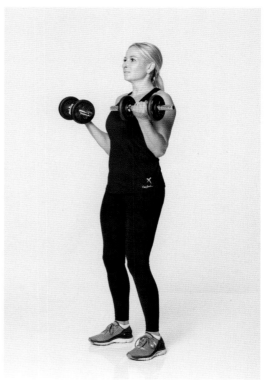

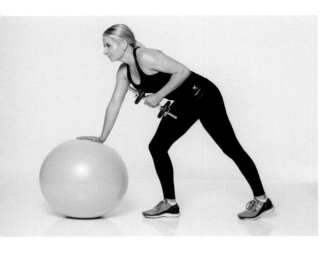

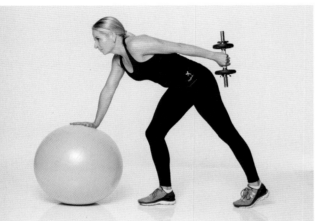

TRICEPS KICKBACKS

This exercise can be done with an exercise ball, a training bench or a low table. Place your right hand on the exercise ball and bend your right leg for support. Leaning forward, make sure your back is straight and your abdominals are tight.

With your left hand holding the dumbbell, bring it up in close to your rib cage keeping your elbow in a fixed position. This is your starting position; from here extend your hand behind you, contracting your triceps muscle, then bring your hand back next to your rib cage. Your upper arm stays in the same place throughout the movement: it's just your lower arm that is moving. Breathe out as your arm extends backwards and breathe in when you bring your hand back in towards your rib cage.

MOUNTAIN CLIMBERS X 20 REPS

Depending upon your level of strength, mountain climbers can be done either on the ground or with hands on an exercise ball. This is a tough exercise but it is fantastic for your core strength.

Mountain Climbers on the ground: Place your hands slightly wider than shoulder-width apart and feet up on toes. Bring one knee into your chest keeping your leg off the ground through the movement then back out to the start. Repeat with the opposite leg for a total of 20 reps (10 reps per leg).

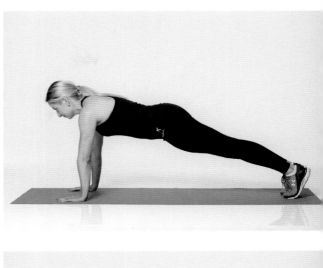

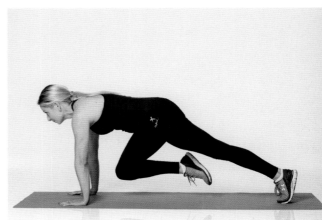

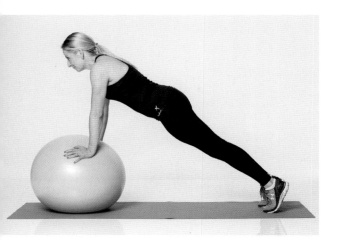

Mountain Climbers on an exercise ball:
Place your hands on top of the exercise ball, slightly to the side, with your feet up on toes. With your abdominals tight, bring one knee in towards your chest and back down to the start position. Repeat with the opposite leg. Breathe out when your leg is contracting in towards you and breathe in when your leg is extending back down to the start position, then repeat with the other leg. This exercise involves balance and concentration, so take your time and don't rush the exercise.

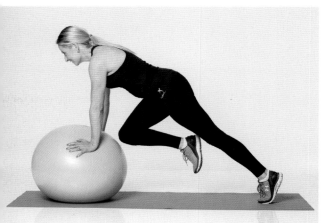

LOWER ABS: INS AND OUTS

This exercise may take a few sessions to master, but stick with it and you will reap the benefits. Sit on the ground with your hands softly supporting you behind your back. Lean back slightly and bring your knees and feet up off the ground. At the same time, extend your feet outwards and lean back a little further, then bring your knees in and come forward, so you are extending out and then crunching back together. Repeat this exercise for 15 reps, having a 60-second rest to recover after each set.

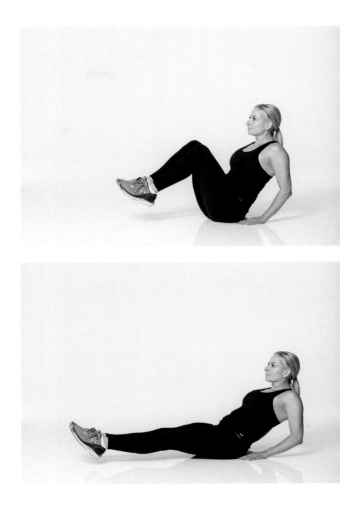

WEIGHTS PROGRAM #2

It is time to ramp up your training and this program will definitely do that! This is also a full-body program, but it is set out in a circuit format. Complete one exercise after another until you get through all of them, then have 60 seconds recovery before repeating the circuit. Do a total of four sets of this circuit with 12 reps of each exercise. This program provides a higher level of intensity and it is a great progression from the first program.

FULL-BODY CIRCUIT

4 SETS / 12 REPS / 60-SECOND RECOVERY BETWEEN CIRCUITS / SPEED 3:0:3

EXERCISES	DATE		DATE		DATE		DATE		DATE		DATE		DATE		DATE	
	REPS	WEIGHT	REPS	WEIGHT	REPS	WEIGHT	REPS	WEIGHT	REPS	WEIGHT	REPS	WEIGHT	REPS	WEIGHT	REPS	WEIGHT
Lunges																
Dumbbell Bent-over Row																
Dumbbell Press on Exercise Ball																
Exercise Ball Wall Squat																
Lying Back Extension																
Lateral Raise																
Elbow to Knee Abdominals																
Prone Hold																

LUNGES

Holding a dumbbell in each hand, stand with your feet shoulder-width apart – pretend you are standing on railway tracks. Step one leg forward and bend the front leg down so that your knee is at a 90-degree angle. Make sure your front knee does NOT go forward over your front toe. The back leg is just there to support you and it should not be carrying any weight. Push up through your front heel (your toes should be in the air in your shoes), continue for 12 reps on one leg and then swap legs. Breathe in on the way down and out on the way up. Keep your abdominals tight and back straight throughout the movement.

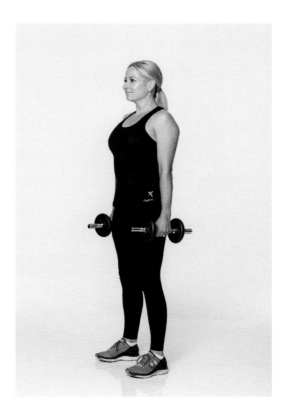
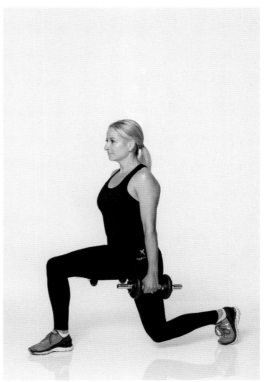

DUMBBELL BENT-OVER ROW

Stand with your feet shoulder-width apart holding dumbbells, with soft, slightly bent knees. Bend forward with your back straight and abdominals tight. Bring the dumbbells up to a 90-degree angle so your elbows are high, in line with your shoulder joint and not making their way backwards. Focus on squeezing between your shoulderblades, then slowly lower hands down towards the ground in a controlled manner and repeat. Breathe out when you bring your hands upwards and breathe in when you lower your hands.

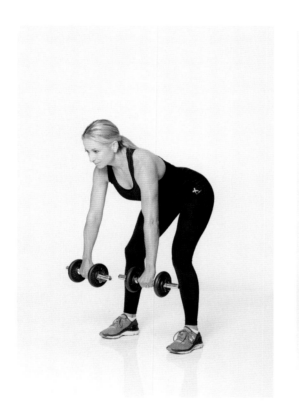
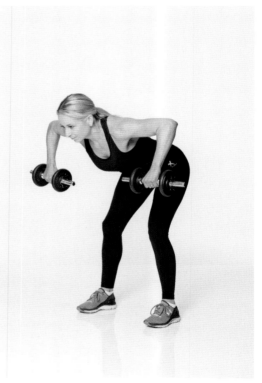

DUMBBELL PRESS ON EXERCISE BALL

Lay your shoulders on your exercise ball (this exercise can also be done on a training bench) and keep your abdominals tight and hips up. Feet are shoulder-width apart. Holding dumbbells with straight arms out in front of your chest, bend your elbows until they get to 90 degrees and then push your arms up straight without locking your elbow joint. Then, slowly go back to 90 degrees to repeat. Keep your abdominals tight throughout the movement to maintain your balance.

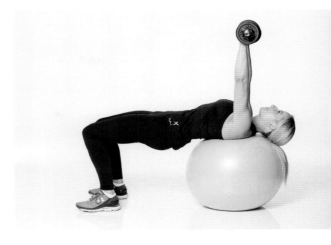

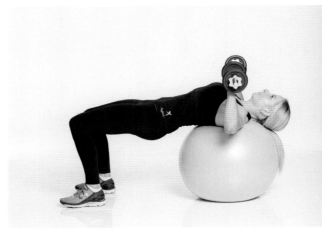

EXERCISE BALL WALL SQUAT

Place the exercise ball against the small of your back while leaning against the wall. Place feet out in front, so when you go into the sitting position your knees are at 90 degrees, with knees not going past your toes. Holding dumbbells, sit down to 90 degrees, then push up through your heels, then slowly back down again (there should be no weight on your toes). Breathe in on the way down and breathe out on the way up. Control the movement, remembering the speed of each rep is 3:0:3; that is, three seconds down and three seconds back up.

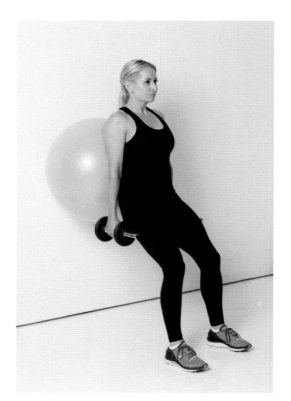
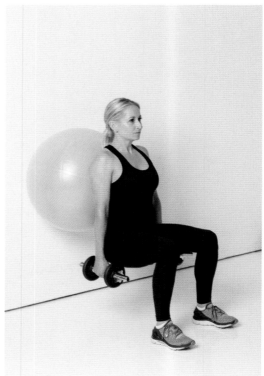

LYING BACK EXTENSION

This exercise looks really simple but is a great one for strengthening your lower back. Lie face down with your arms and legs outstretched on the floor. Simultaneously, bring both arms, head and both legs up off the floor and hold for two seconds, then gently lower back to the floor and repeat. Breathe out on the way up and breathe in on the way back to the floor.

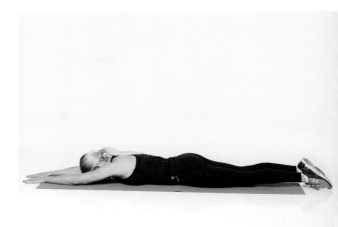

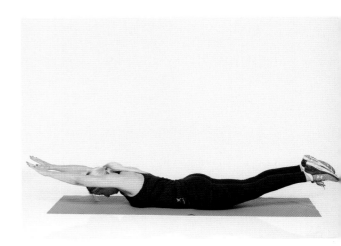

LATERAL RAISE

Stand tall with feet shoulder-width apart and soft knees. Holding dumbbells, slowly bring your arms out to the sides, so your hands are just slightly lower than your shoulder joints and your elbow joints are slightly bent. Then lower your arms very slowly back down, without taking the tension out of the movement when you get to the bottom. Keep the movement going and repeat. Make sure your abdominals are switched on throughout the whole movement.

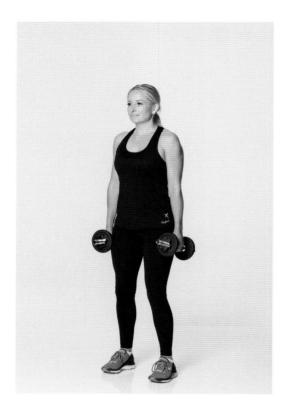
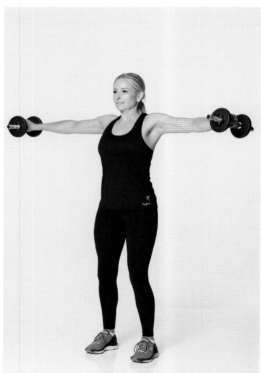

ABDOMINALS: ELBOWS TO KNEES X 20 REPS

Lie on the floor with your hands behind your head and bring your knees up so your knee joint is at 90 degrees. Simultaneously, bring one knee up and across your body to reach the opposite elbow, while your other leg is outstretched, keep both legs off the ground through the movement. Then, lower back down without your head touching the floor until your knees are back to the starting position. Repeat with the opposite leg and opposite elbow. Complete 20 reps (10 on each side).

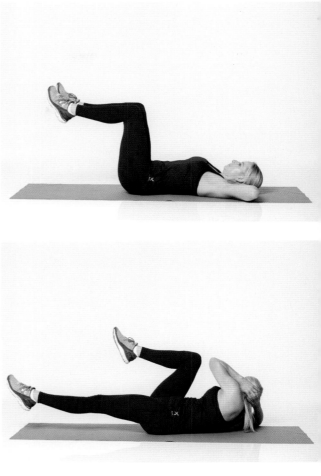

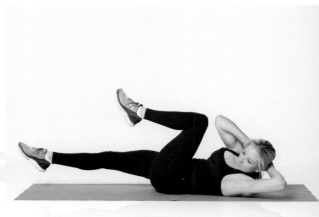

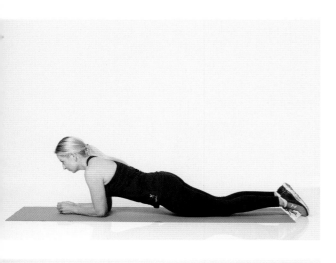

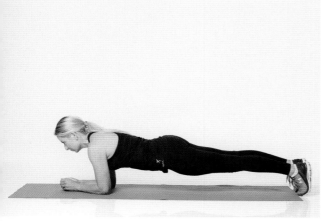

PRONE HOLD X 60 SECONDS

This is a great exercise to improve your core strength. It takes focus and control, but it is totally worth it. There are three progressions of this exercise depending on your level. Start on your knees and, once your strength improves, you can progress to the more advanced versions of the exercise.

Prone hold on knees: Lie face down on the floor supported by your elbows and up on your knees. Ensure your elbows are directly under your shoulder joints. Keep your back flat so it is not dipping too far towards the floor and make sure your bottom is not sticking up in the air. Once you have your position, focus on bringing your belly button into your spine and hold it there while you continue to breathe normally. Hold this position for 60 seconds.

Prone hold on toes: Lie face down on the floor supported by your elbows and up on your toes. Ensure your elbows are directly under your shoulder joints. Keep your back flat so it is not dipping too far towards the floor and make sure your bottom is not sticking up in the air. Once you have your position, focus on bringing your belly button into your spine and hold it there while you continue to breathe normally. Hold this position for 60 seconds. If at any time you feel your lower back hurting, this could mean one of two things: you need to lift your bottom up a little bit higher, or your core is not yet strong enough for this exercise, so revert back to your knees.

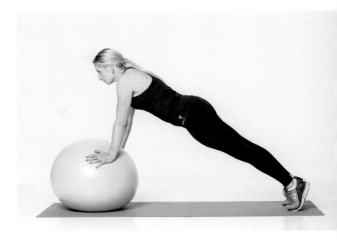

Prone hold on your exercise ball: Place your hands on top and slightly to the sides of the exercise ball. You should have a slight bend in your elbow joint. Your feet are up on your toes. Ensure your hands are directly under your shoulder joints. Keep your back flat so that it is not dipping too far towards the floor and make sure your bottom is not sticking up in the air. Once you have your position, focus on bringing your belly button into your spine and holding it there while you continue to breathe normally. Hold this position for 60 seconds. This is a great core exercise that will quickly tell you whether or not you are ready for it. Your balance is directly related to your core, so if you try this exercise and can't seem to control the ball and keep it still, or if your lower back starts to hurt, stick with the prone hold on toes until your core gets a little stronger.

Congratulations on getting through both programs! If you find yourself wanting more after completing these two four-week programs, I suggest you contact a personal trainer or check out my website www.kimbeach.com to help take your weight training to the next level.

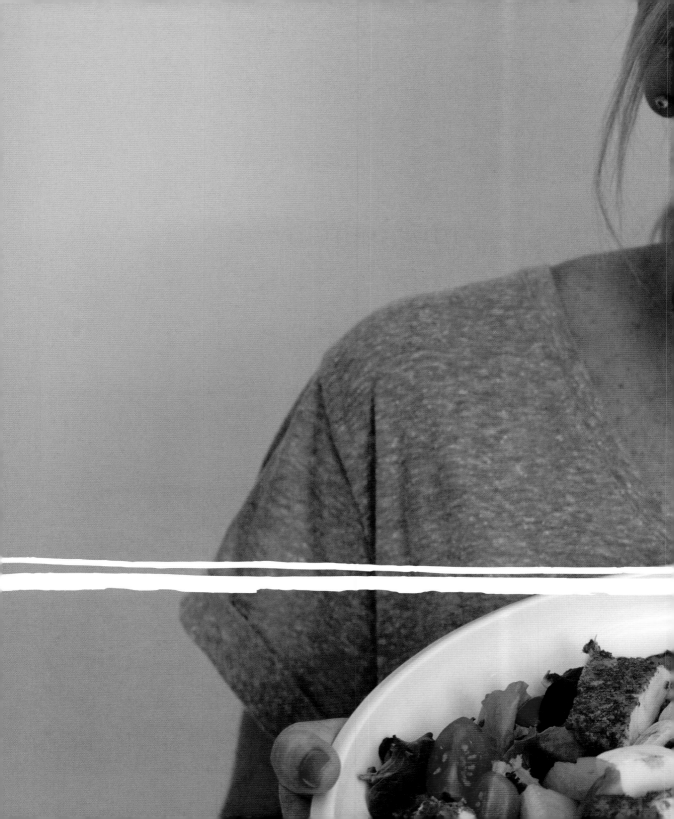

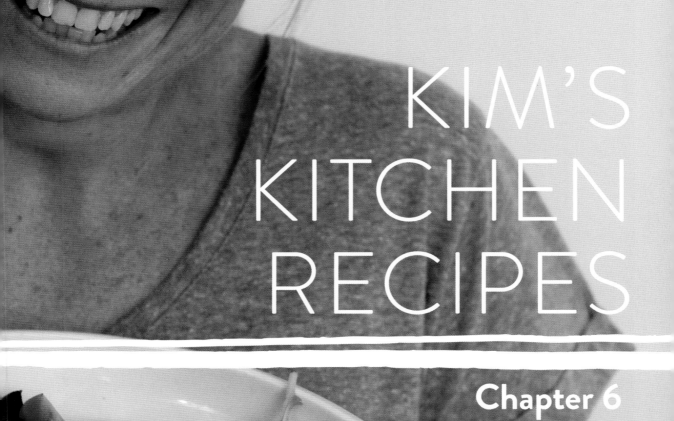

KIM'S
KITCHEN
RECIPES

Chapter 6

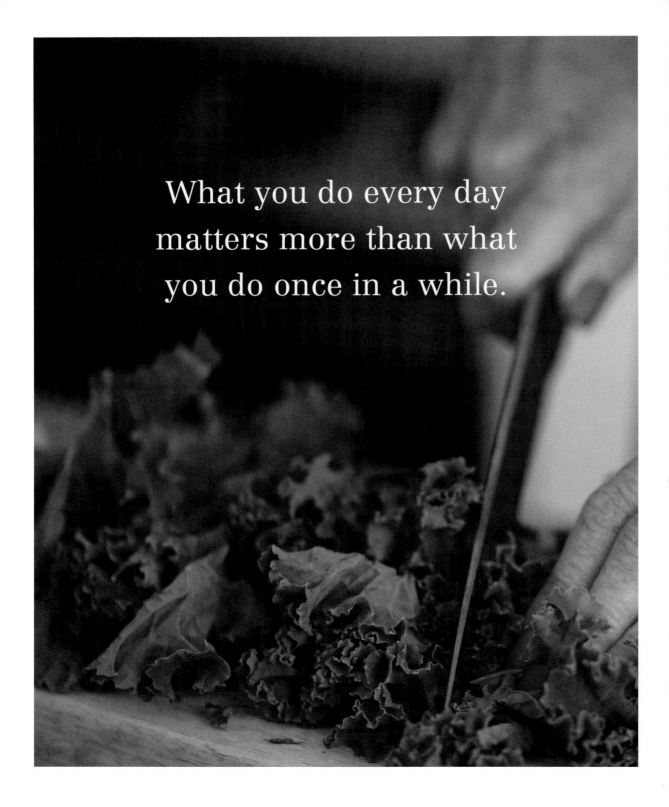

As with my approach to training and nutrition, I like to keep my recipes simple. Most of these recipes can be prepared and cooked in less than 20 minutes. They are all designed around pairing the right macronutrients together at the right times of day, as follows:

Meal 1 = Breakfast	Carbohydrates + Protein
Meal 2 = Morning Tea	Carbohydrates + Protein
Meal 3 = Lunch	Carbohydrates + Protein
Meal 4 = Afternoon Tea	Good Fats + Protein
Meal 5 = Dinner	Good Fats + Protein
Meal 6 = Treats	Around 1–2 times per week

TIP: *Remember, a sandwich press is your best friend when it comes to preparing many of these meals. Lots of these recipes were prepared in my very own kitchen using my trusty sandwich press, which I take with me everywhere, even when I travel. The press can be used with the lid down to cook things on both sides quickly, or as a flat griddle with the lid up. The press is so quick and simple to use and, even more importantly, super-easy to clean! (If you don't have a sandwich press, use a non-stick frying pan instead.)*

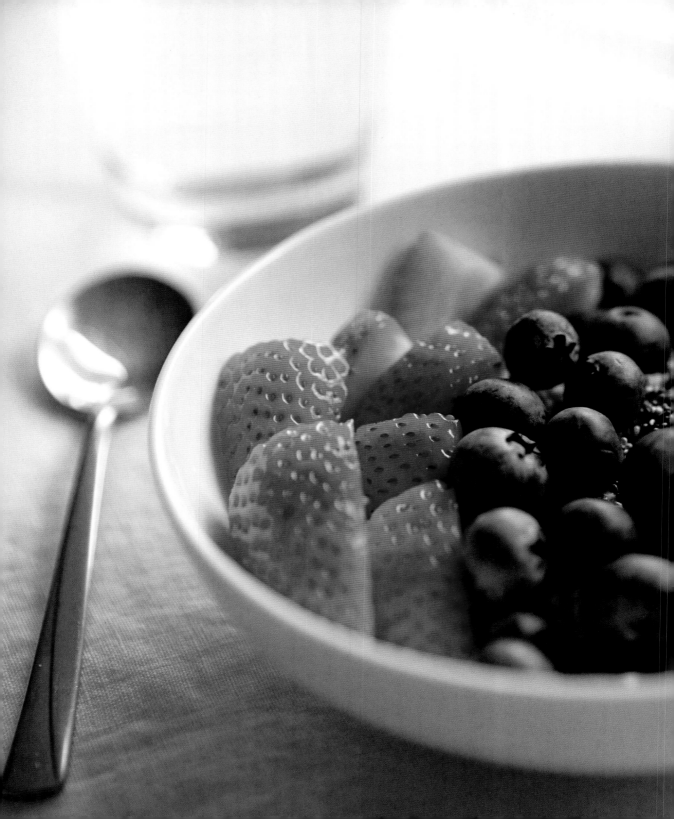

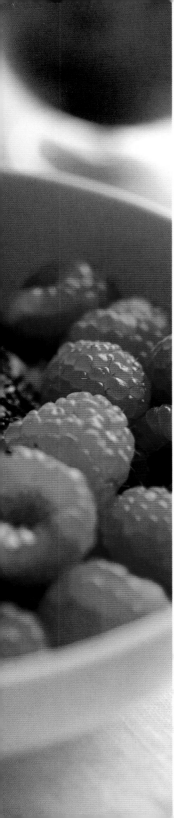

OATS & BERRIES

This is definitely my favourite breakfast!

SERVES 1

½ cup (50g) oats
½ tsp cinnamon
½ cup (125ml) rice milk
½ tsp chia seeds
½ cup (70g) mixed berries (frozen is fine)

Put the oats in a colander and give them a good rinse, then drain excess water. Transfer oats to a bowl, along with the cinnamon and milk. Cover with plastic wrap and stand in the fridge overnight. In the morning, top the oats with chia seeds and berries.

> **NOTE:** *Cinnamon is a great spice to help keep your blood-sugar levels stable and it's also a delicious way to add sweetness to any dish. When it comes to oats, it is always a good idea to give them a good rinse before preparing to soften them up so they are easier to digest. If you are cooking your oats as porridge they will expand and double in size, so you may only want to cook ¼ cup, which will turn into ½ cup once cooked.*

BIG BREAKFAST SAUSAGE

MAKES 8, SERVES 4

500g pork, turkey or chicken mince
2 spring onions, finely chopped
1 tsp garlic powder
1 tbsp pure maple syrup
1 tsp smoked paprika

1 tbsp chopped dill
4 thin slices sweet potato
1 cup (45g) spinach leaves
About 6 button mushrooms, chopped

Turn the sandwich press on and preheat the oven to 180°C. Line a baking tray with foil. Put the mince in a big bowl, add the spring onions, garlic, maple syrup, smoked paprika, dill, and season with salt and pepper. Mix until well combined. Using your hands, form mixture into sausages. Lay the sausages on the baking tray and bake for 10–12 minutes until cooked, turning once.

When the sausages are cooked, lay the sweet potato in the sandwich press and cook with the lid down for about 30 seconds. Transfer to a plate, then put the mushrooms and spinach in the sandwich press and warm through. Plate up and enjoy!

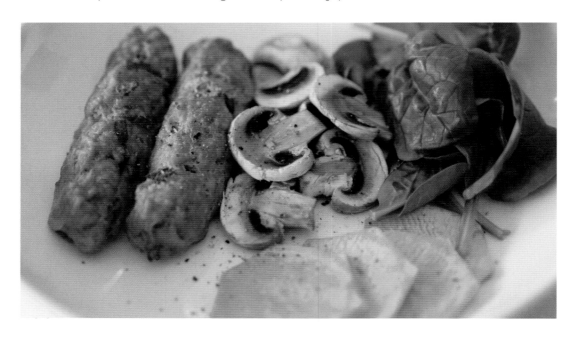

BREAKFAST SCRAMBLE

SERVES 1

2 tsp olive oil

2 eggwhites

½ cup (70g) grated sweet potato

2 tsp low-fat cottage cheese

1 slice turkey breast, chopped

1 tsp chopped chives

Heat the oil in a small frying pan on medium heat. Add the remaining ingredients and stir constantly for about 5 minutes, until the eggwhites start to cook through. Plate up and enjoy!

NOTE: *You can add cayenne pepper for a little heat in this dish.*

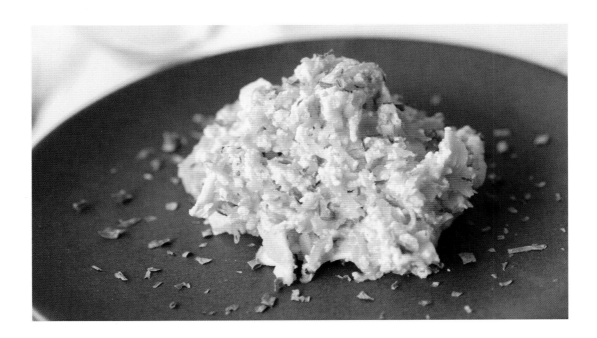

FRENCH TOAST

SERVES 1

2 eggwhites

1 tsp cinnamon

2 slices rye bread

1–2 tsps low-fat cottage cheese

½ cup (70g) raspberries (frozen is fine)

Rice malt syrup, for drizzling

Preheat the sandwich press or use a non-stick frying pan. Mix eggwhites and cinnamon together. Soak bread in the eggwhite mixture so that both sides are covered, then place on sandwich press and cook with lid up for 2–3 minutes.

Place French toast on a plate and dollop with cottage cheese, scatter with raspberries and drizzle with rice malt syrup.

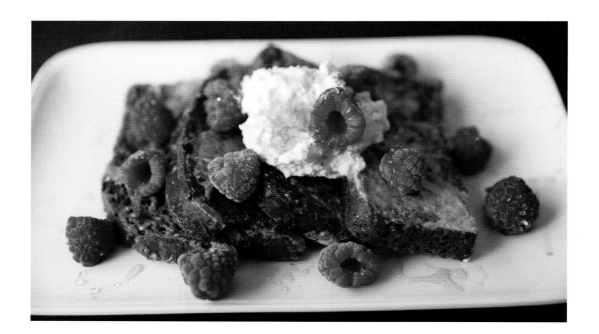

BREKKY SMOOTHIE

SERVES 1

½ cup (50g) oats
½ cup (70g) frozen mixed berries
1 small frozen banana

1 cup (250ml) rice milk, or milk of your choice
1 tsp chia seeds
½ tsp ground cinnamon

Put all of the ingredients into a blender, blend until smooth and serve.

NOTE: *Optional – add a scoop of vanilla protein powder to the smoothie. This will not only increase the protein, it will also add a little more sweetness.*

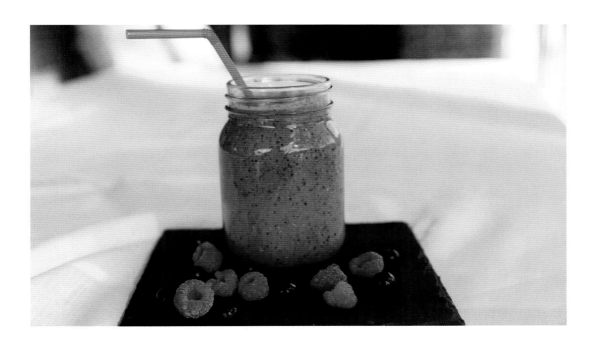

QUINOA BREKKY BOWL

SERVES 2

½ cup (100g) quinoa
1 tsp ground cinnamon, plus extra for sprinkling
¼ cup (65g) unsweetened apple sauce
¼ cup (60ml) rice milk, or milk of your choice (optional)
¼ cup (60g) Greek-style yoghurt
½ cup (70g) raspberries

Put the quinoa in a small saucepan with 1½ cups of water, the cinnamon and apple sauce. Bring to the boil, then cover and reduce to low heat, simmering for 10 minutes or until liquid has been soaked up.

Transfer the mixture to a serving bowl (with milk, if using). Add a dollop of yoghurt, sprinkle with extra cinnamon and dress with raspberries.

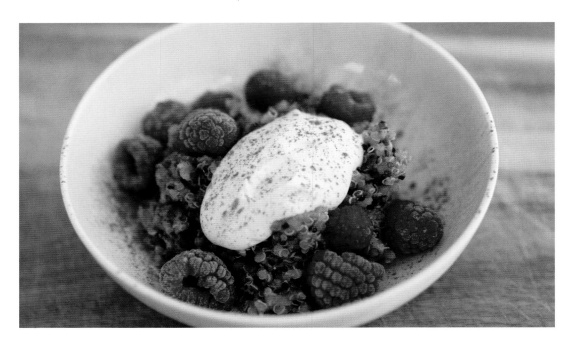

KIM'S RYE TOAST

SERVES 1

1 slice rye bread
2 tsp low-fat cottage cheese
1 slice turkey breast
2 cherry tomatoes, sliced

Toast the bread in a toaster. Spread with the cottage cheese, add turkey and tomatoes, and season with salt and pepper.

NOTE: *This is a breakfast high in protein and full of fibre that is quick and easy to prepare.*

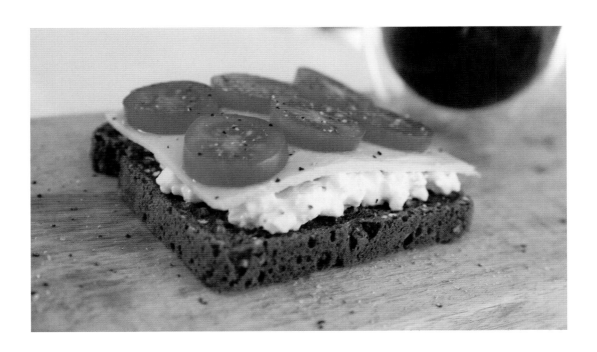

CHOCONANA PANCAKES

SERVES 1

2 eggwhites
¼ cup (25g) rolled oats, rinsed and drained
½ scoop chocolate protein powder
1 banana

Rice malt syrup (or your favourite natural sweetener), for drizzling
½ cup (70g) of blueberries (or similar) for garnishing

Preheat the sandwich press or use a non-stick frying pan. In a medium bowl, combine the eggwhites, oats and protein powder. Mash three-quarters of the banana with a fork and add it to the bowl. Mix the ingredients together and pour onto the sandwich press with the lid up or into the frying pan, cooking for 2 minutes each side. When done, place the pancakes on a plate, dress with slices of the remaining banana and berries, and drizzle rice malt syrup over the top.

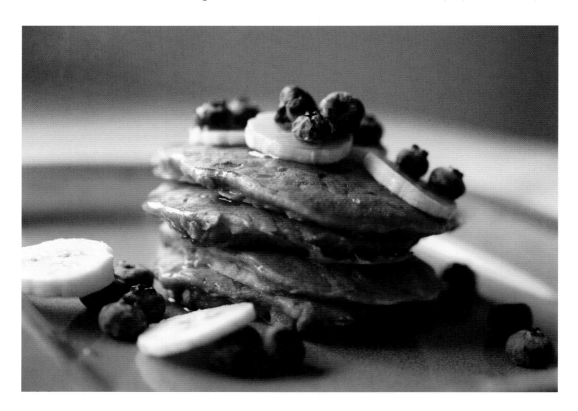

SWEET POTATO & CAULIFLOWER FRITTERS

SERVES 1

1 zucchini, grated
½ cup (70g) grated sweet potato
½ cup (60g) finely chopped cauliflower

½ cup (50g) grated parmesan cheese
2 eggwhites

Preheat the sandwich press or use a non-stick frying pan. Put the zucchini into a colander and press with the back of a spoon to remove excess moisture, or squeeze with your hands. Mix all of the ingredients together, season with salt and pepper and spoon onto the sandwich press into small fritters. Cook with the lid up for 5 minutes on each side.

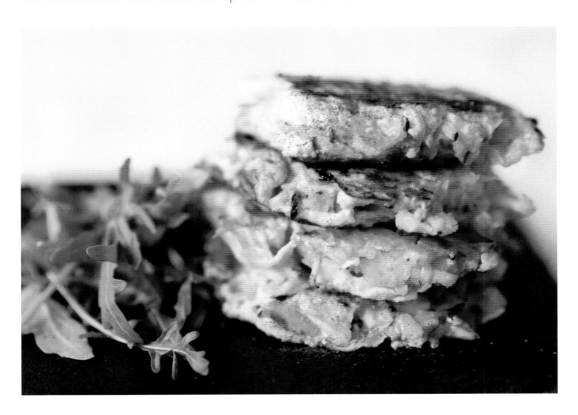

CARROT CAKE BALLS

MAKES 8–10 BALLS (2 BALLS PER SERVE)

1 cup (95g) rolled oats
1 cup (25g) puffed rice
1 carrot, grated
6 dates, chopped

1 tsp vanilla essence
1 tsp ground cinnamon
1 tsp chia seeds
1 tbsp rice milk, or your milk of choice

Put the oats, puffed rice, carrot, date, vanilla essence, cinnamon and chia seeds into a food processor and blend until combined. Add the rice milk and blend to a smooth paste.

Use your hands to form the mixture into balls (a bit smaller than a golf ball) and place balls on a tray in the fridge. Allow to set for at least 1 hour.

Store balls in an airtight container in the fridge. These are a great option for when you are on the go.

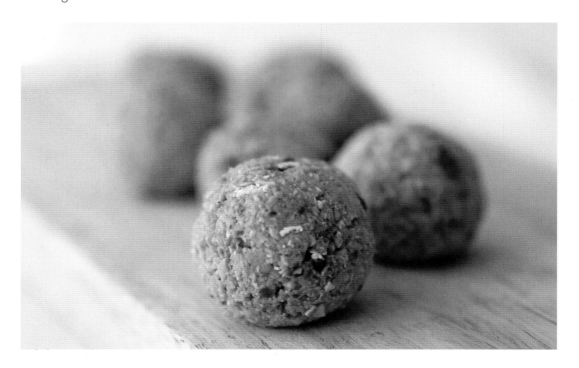

SPICY CHEESE DIP

SERVES 1

½ cup (125g) low-fat cottage cheese
1 tsp smoked paprika
½ tsp ground turmeric
½ tsp onion powder

½ tsp garlic powder
½ tsp cayenne pepper
1 carrot, cut into sticks
1 celery stalk, cut into sticks

Put the cottage cheese, smoked paprika, turmeric, onion powder, garlic powder and cayenne pepper into a small blender and season with salt and pepper. Blend until smooth and creamy.

Transfer dip to a small bowl and serve with carrot and celery sticks.

NOTE: *This is a great option to make ahead and take out with you; a bit of spice to get your metabolism firing and also to curb your hunger.*

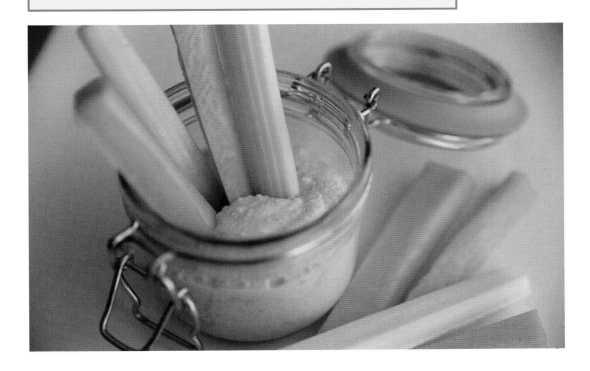

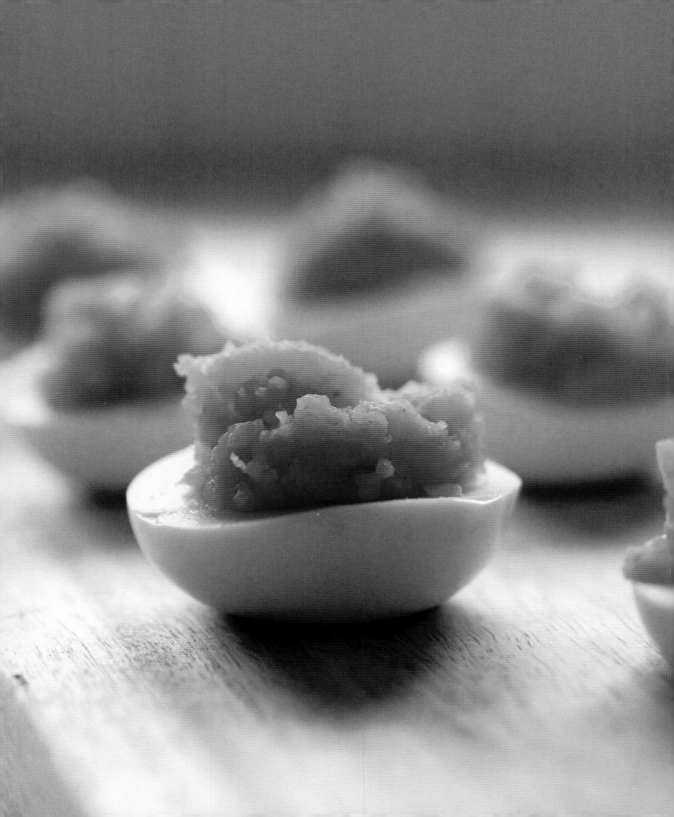

SWEET POTATO DEVILLED EGGS

SERVES 2

4 eggs
1 small sweet potato
1 tsp smoked paprika
½ tsp curry powder

Put the eggs into a medium saucepan and add water to cover. Cook over high heat for 10 minutes, or until eggs are hard boiled.

Peel the sweet potato and chop into 2cm cubes. Steam sweet potato in a vegetable steamer or double boiler until soft. Transfer to a bowl, mash with a fork, than add smoked paprika and curry powder, season with salt and pepper, then mix well to combine.

Remove shell from eggs, cut in half and remove yolk. With a teaspoon, spoon the sweet potato mixture into the hollow eggwhites and enjoy.

> **NOTE:** *If you have any sweet potato left over, store it in an airtight container in the fridge. It will last at least a week. Sweet potato is a great source of carbohydrate.*

CINNAMON APPLES

SERVES 1

1 apple
½ cup (125g) Greek-style yoghurt
½ tsp ground cinnamon

Slice the apple into eight slices. In a small bowl, mix yoghurt and cinnamon together. Dollop the yoghurt mixture onto apple slices and enjoy.

NOTE: *This is an easy snack that is high in protein and fibre. The cinnamon is there to help stabilise your blood-sugar levels.*

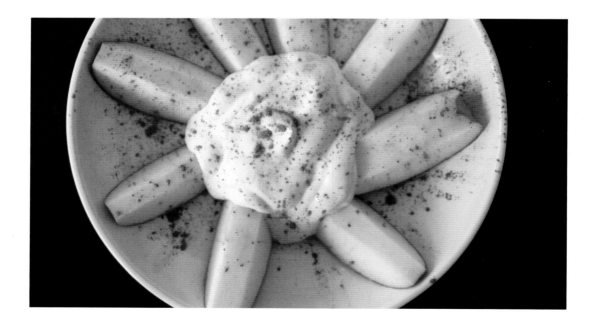

CELERY BOATS

This is one of my favourite go-to snacks: I love this combo!

SERVES 1

2 celery stalks
½ cup (125g) low-fat cottage cheese
1 tsp yeast-extract spread
½ tsp chia seeds

Wash celery and cut the ends of the stalks on an angle so you have a nice boat shape.

In a small bowl, combine cottage cheese, the spread and chia seeds.

Spoon the mixture into celery boats and enjoy.

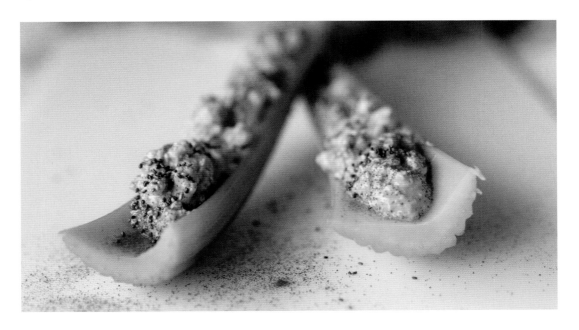

TURKEY WRAPS

SERVES 1

½ cup cooked quinoa

2 tsp crumbled feta cheese

3 thin strips of capsicum, chopped into tiny squares

2 slices turkey breast, cut into strips

Mix quinoa, feta and capsicum together. Lay both slices of turkey out flat, side by side. Spoon mixture onto both, wrap each one into a cylinder and enjoy.

NOTE: *When you cook quinoa it doubles in size so, if you want a serving of ½ cup, use ¼ cup of raw quinoa.*

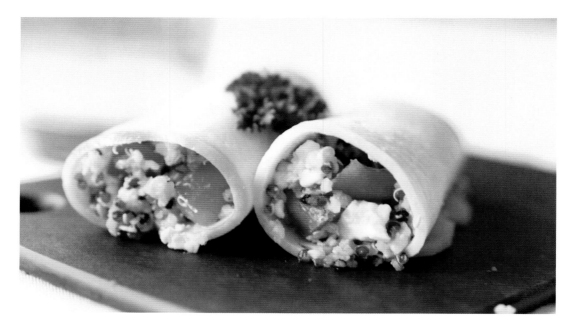

BLACK BEAN DIP WITH VEGIE STICKS

SERVES 1

½ cup (115g) tinned refried black beans
3 thin strips capsicum, plus extra for garnish
1 tsp smoked paprika
½ tsp curry powder

½ tsp cayenne pepper (optional)
2 tsp apple cider vinegar
1 carrot
1 cucumber

Put the black beans, capsicum, smoked paprika, curry powder, cayenne pepper and apple cider vinegar into a food processor and process until smooth.

Slice carrot and cucumber into sticks.

Spoon dip into a small bowl and serve on a plate surrounded by vegie dipping sticks.

NOTE: *This tasty morning tea is a good source of carbohydrate as well as being high in protein and fibre: exactly what you want!*

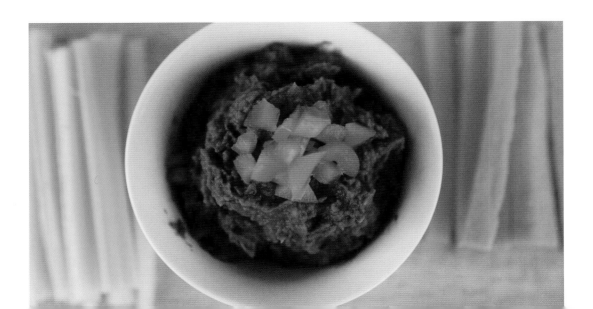

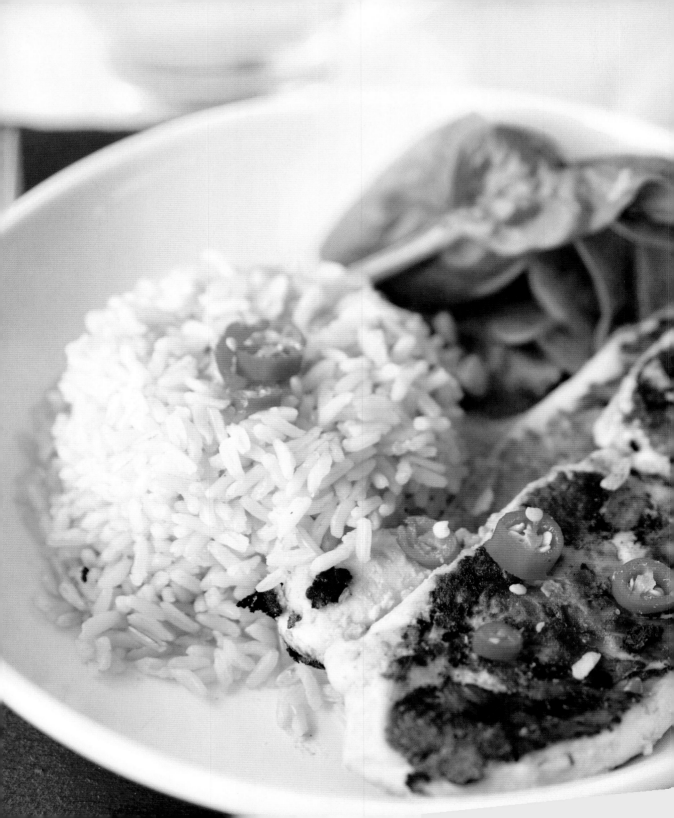

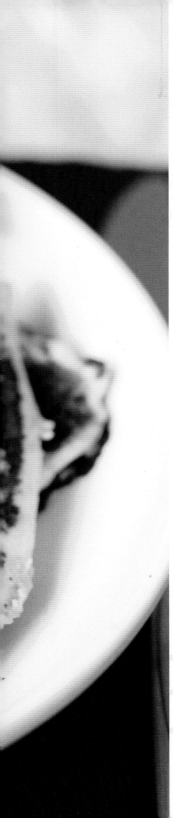

SWEET MUSTARD CHICKEN SALAD

SERVES 1

¼ cup (60g) English mustard
1 tbsp rice malt syrup
1 tsp smoked paprika
½ tsp garlic powder
2 chicken tenderloins
½ cup cooked brown rice
½ cup (25g) baby spinach leaves
1 fresh chilli, finely sliced

In a bowl, combine the mustard, rice malt syrup, smoked paprika and garlic powder, and season with salt and pepper. Give it a good stir, then add the chicken and coat well.

Preheat the sandwich press and cook the chicken with the lid down for about 4 minutes (alternatively, cook the chicken for about 4 minutes on each side in a non-stick frying pan). Set aside on a board to rest.

Place the chicken, rice and spinach leaves on your plate and top with the chilli.

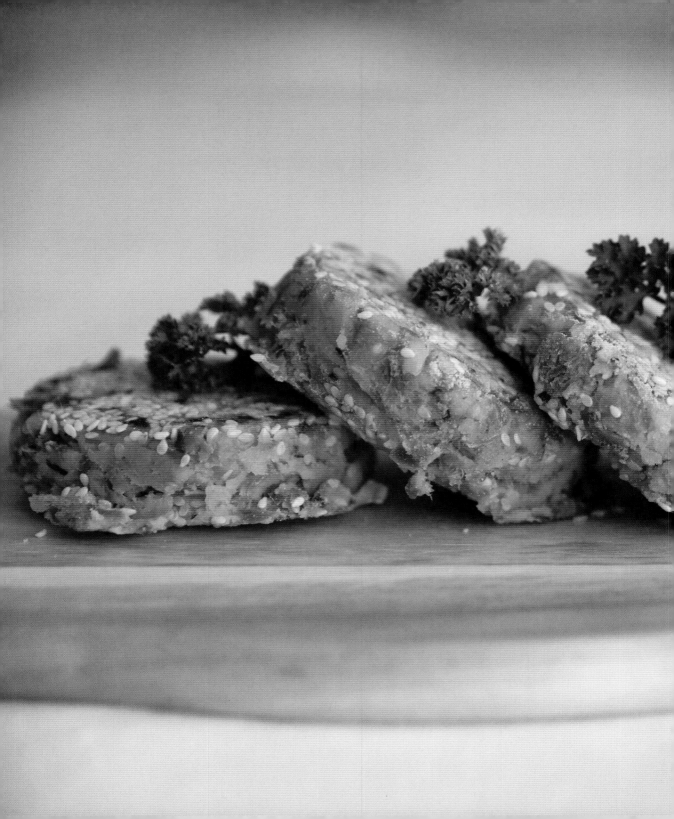

TUNA AND SWEET POTATO PATTIES

These are great to cook up and have ready for the week ahead. They taste even better the next day too.

SERVES 4

2 small sweet potatoes (about 500g)
1 tbsp olive oil
4 spring onions, finely sliced
1–2 garlic cloves, grated or chopped
400g can tuna in spring water, drained

1 egg, lightly beaten
1 cup (80g) rice crumbs
1 tsp finely chopped flat-leaf parsley
2 tbsp spelt flour
2 tsp sesame seeds

Preheat the sandwich press. Cut the sweet potato into small cubes and steam them for 5–10 minutes until soft. Transfer to a bowl and use a fork to mash roughly.

Heat olive oil in a non-stick frying pan over medium heat, add the spring onions and garlic and cook for a couple of minutes until softened. Add the tuna, sweet potato, egg, rice crumbs and parsley to mixture. Stir until combined. Use your hands to form mixture into patties. Combine the flour and sesame seeds in a bowl, and lightly coat each patty (dusting off any excess). Place patties on the sandwich press and, with the lid up, cook on each side for 4 minutes until warmed through and golden.

> **NOTE:** *I use egg rings and place a patty in each one while cooking, so they all come out the same size. You can use a bit of olive oil spray on the sandwich press to give them that nice golden colour.*

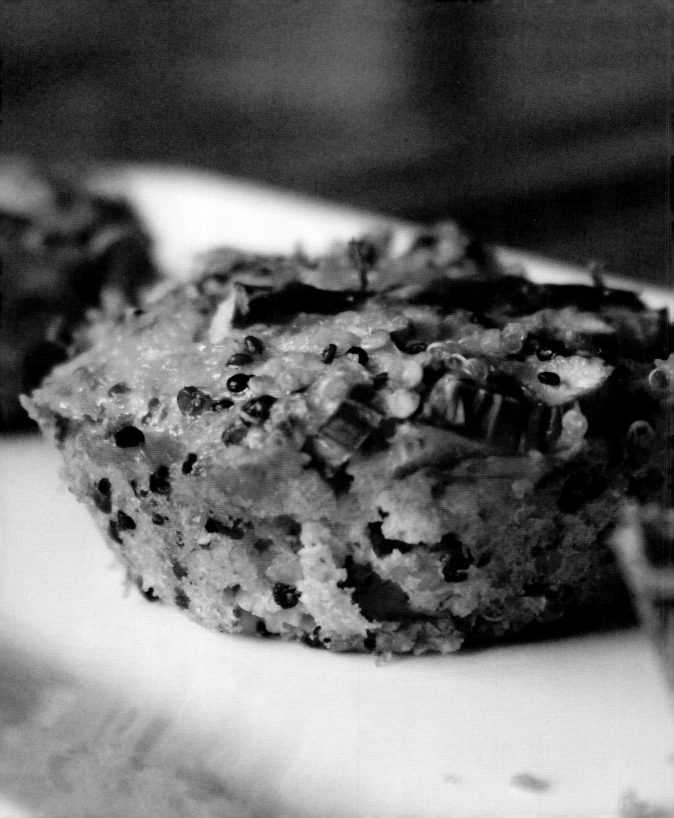

QUINOA AND ASPARAGUS MUFFINS

This is a really tasty recipe to make as you prep for the week ahead.

MAKES 6 MUFFINS; SERVES 3

Olive oil spray, for greasing
½ cup (100g) uncooked quinoa
1 bunch asparagus
½ cup (50g) grated parmesan cheese

2 garlic cloves, crushed
2 eggs
1 tsp smoked paprika
½ tsp cayenne pepper

Preheat the oven to 180°C. Lightly grease a muffin tin with olive oil spray.

Put the quinoa in a medium saucepan with 1½ cups of water, bring to the boil then reduce heat to low and cover. Stir every couple of minutes to prevent the quinoa sticking to the saucepan. Once all liquid has been absorbed, the quinoa is ready. Set aside to cool.

Cut the tips off the asparagus and reserve for decorating the top of muffins. Break off the ends of the asparagus stalks to remove the hard chalky bits. Thinly slice the asparagus into small discs.

In a bowl, combine the quinoa, asparagus, parmesan, garlic, eggs, smoked paprika and cayenne pepper, and season with salt. Mix well, then spoon into the muffin tins. Add an asparagus tip on top of each muffin. Place in the oven for 20 minutes or until cooked and lightly brown.

> **NOTE:** *Quinoa doubles in size when it is cooked, so this recipe yields 1 cup of cooked quinoa.*

CHICKEN NUGGETS

SERVES 2

4 chicken tenderloins
1 egg
½ cup (100g) teff

1 tsp smoked paprika
½ tsp curry powder
½ tsp garlic powder

Preheat the oven to 180°C. Line a baking tray with baking paper.

Slice the chicken tenderloins into small nugget-size pieces (3 or 4 pieces per tenderloin). In a small bowl, whisk the egg to make an egg wash. In a separate bowl, combine the teff, smoked paprika, curry powder and garlic powder, and mix together.

Dip the chicken pieces into the egg wash, then into the teff mixture and coat well. Lay the nuggets on the prepared tray and bake for 15 minutes, turning once. Serve with salad.

NOTE: *Teff is gluten free, high in protein and a great source of carbohydrate. It is the world's smallest grain – and so versatile to work with!*

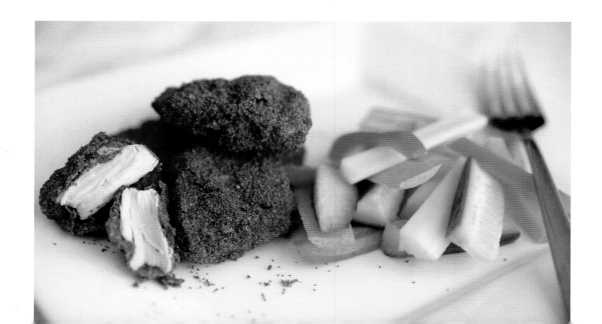

CREAMY BROCCOLI SOUP

This soup is so creamy and delicious!

SERVES 2

Olive oil, for frying
1 garlic clove, crushed
1 onion, chopped
1 broccoli head, chopped into florets

¼ cauliflower head, chopped into florets
¼ cup (50g) teff
2 cups (500ml) chicken stock
¼ cup low-fat cottage cheese

In a non-stick frying pan, add a dash of olive oil, the garlic and onion and sauté until onion is translucent. Add the broccoli, cauliflower, teff and stock, season with salt and pepper and bring to the boil, then cover and simmer for 10 minutes.

Transfer the cooked ingredients to a blender and process until smooth. Add the cottage cheese and blend again. Put the mixture in a saucepan, heat through and serve. Garnish with your favourite herbs and spices, if desired.

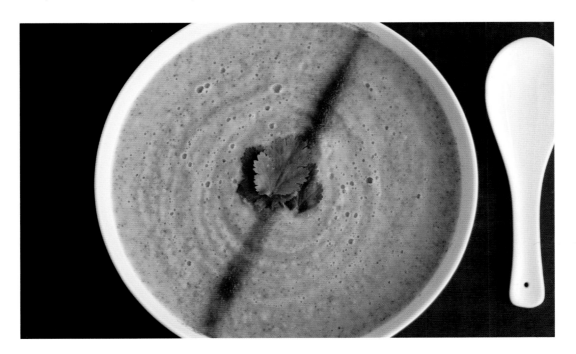

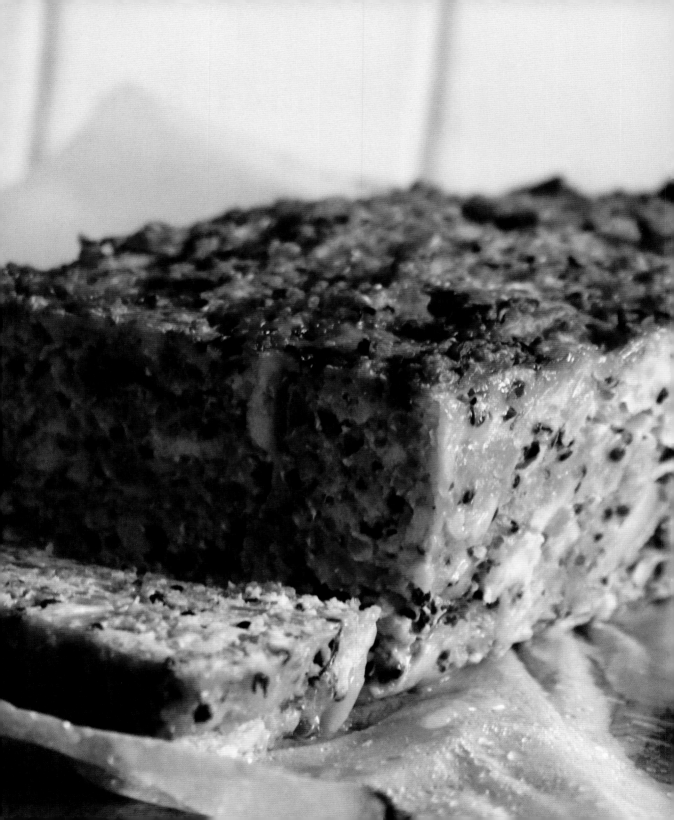

CHICKEN AND QUINOA MEATLOAF

SERVES 4

½ cup (100g) uncooked quinoa
1½ cups (375ml) chicken stock
500g chicken mince
½ cup (40g) mushrooms, chopped
2 garlic cloves, crushed
1 onion, chopped

¾ cup (60g) rice crumbs
2 tbsp tamari (gluten-free soy sauce)
2 tbsp pure maple syrup
1 zucchini, grated
1 carrot, grated
1 egg

Preheat the oven to 180°C. Line a loaf tin with baking paper.

Put quinoa in a small saucepan with the chicken stock. Bring to the boil, then cover and simmer for 10 minutes, stirring occasionally, until all the liquid has been absorbed. Remove from heat and allow to cool.

Combine quinoa with all of the remaining ingredients in a large bowl and mix well. Pour into the prepared loaf tin, flatten the top with a fork and bake for 45 minutes or until cooked (the juices will run clear when you cut into the top).

NOTE: *This is a great recipe to make on a weekend for the week ahead.*

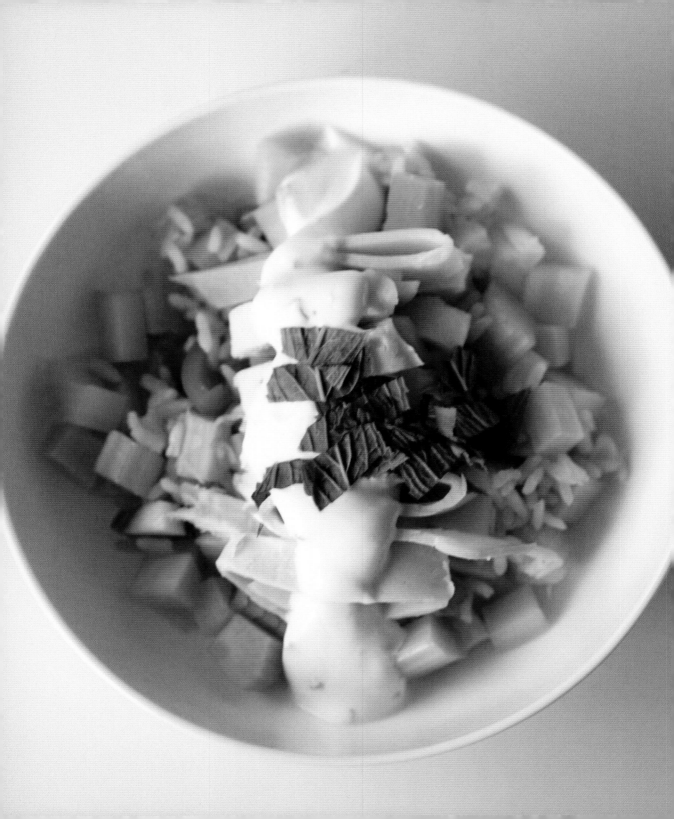

CRUNCHY TURKEY SALAD

A really simple salad that is full of texture and taste!

SERVES 1

¼ cup (45g) brown rice
1 celery stalk
1 carrot
4 cherry tomatoes, quartered
2 thin slices turkey breast, cut into strips
Finely chopped mint leaves, to garnish

DRESSING
⅓ cup (90g) Greek-style yoghurt
1 tsp fresh coriander, finely chopped
2 tsp lemon juice

Cook brown rice according to packet instructions, remembering that one quarter of a cup of uncooked rice will double in size and become half a cup of cooked rice. Transfer to a bowl and allow to cool slightly. If you have precooked your brown rice and it is stored in the fridge, spoon half a cup into a colander, rinse under hot water and transfer it to a bowl.

Chop celery and carrot into small pieces, to add crunch and colour to the salad.

To make the dressing, in a small bowl, combine the yoghurt, coriander and lemon juice, season with salt and pepper and give it a good mix.

In a bowl, combine the celery, carrot and tomato with the rice and mix. Top with turkey and dressing. Garnish with mint.

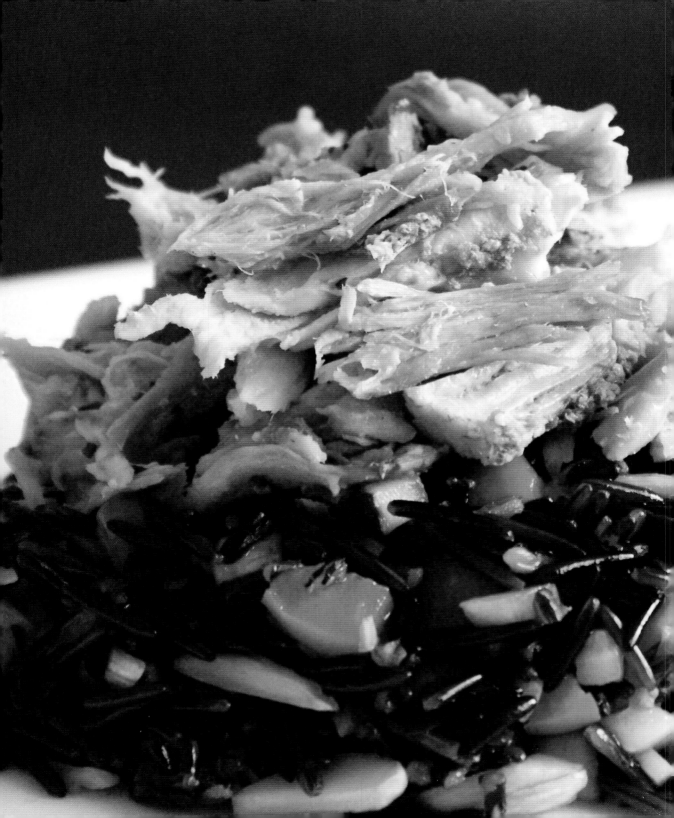

SPICY PULLED PORK WITH WILD RICE

SERVES 4

Slow-cooked pulled pork
2–3kg pork shoulder
1 tsp smoked paprika
1 tsp curry powder
1 tsp turmeric
1 tsp oregano
1 tsp salt
1 tsp pepper
½ tsp cayenne pepper

1 tbsp pure maple syrup
1 onion, thinly sliced
Black wild rice
Olive oil spray
4 garlic cloves, crushed
8 spring onions, finely sliced
2 red capsicum, deseeded and chopped
⅓ cup (40g) slivered almonds
2 cups cooked wild rice

For the pulled pork

Remove any excess fat from the pork. In a bowl, combine smoked paprika, curry powder, turmeric, oregano, salt, pepper and cayenne pepper. Add maple syrup until the rub becomes sticky. Spoon or brush marinade all over pork. Lay the onion in the bottom of a slow-cooker bowl. Place the pork on top, put the lid on and cook on low heat for 6–8 hours. Once cooked, transfer to a plate and let it rest for 10 minutes, then you can start pulling it apart to serve. Pull pork off the bone using two forks and store any leftovers for 3–4 days in an airtight container in the fridge.

For the wild rice

Spray a frying pan with olive oil and heat over medium heat. Add the garlic, spring onions, capsicum and almonds, and stir-fry until all ingredients are warmed through. Add to wild rice in a bowl and mix.

Place rice in a bowl and top with a serving of pulled pork about the size of your fist.

NORI WRAPS

SERVES 1

2 chicken tenderloins
1 tsp smoked paprika
1 tsp curry powder
2 nori sheets

¼ avocado, sliced thinly
6 thin strips capsicum
½ Lebanese (short) cucumber, cut into strips

Preheat the sandwich press or use a non-stick frying pan. Sprinkle chicken with smoked paprika and curry powder on both sides. Lay the chicken on the hot sandwich press and press lid down for 4 minutes or until cooked (or cook for 4 minutes on each side in a non-stick frying pan).

Lay nori sheets out flat and top with chicken, avocado, capsicum and cucumber.
Wrap and enjoy.

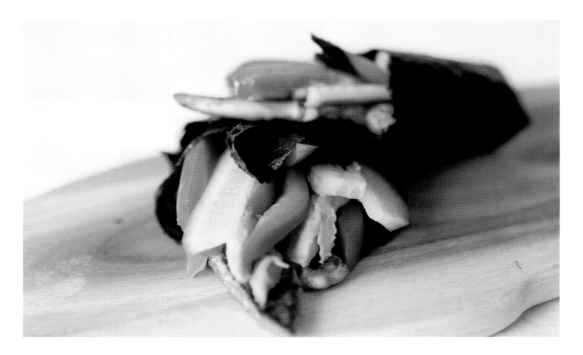

SEED BAR

SERVES 4

¼ cup (60ml) coconut oil

1 tbsp cacao powder

2 tsp pure maple syrup

1 tsp vanilla essence

Pinch of salt

½ cup (60g) slivered almonds

¼ cup (70g) pepitas (pumpkin seeds)

¼ cup (40g) sesame seeds

1 tbsp chia seeds

1 tbsp cacao nibs

1 tsp ground cinnamon

½ cup (40g) desiccated coconut

Line a loaf tin with baking paper. In a small saucepan, heat the coconut oil, cacao, maple syrup, vanilla and salt over medium heat until melted and combined. Remove from the heat. Add the almonds, pepitas, sesame seeds, chia seeds, cacao nibs, cinnamon and coconut. Stir well and pour into a loaf tin. Use the back of a teaspoon to spread the mixture evenly and transfer to the fridge to set for at least an hour. Cut into bars.

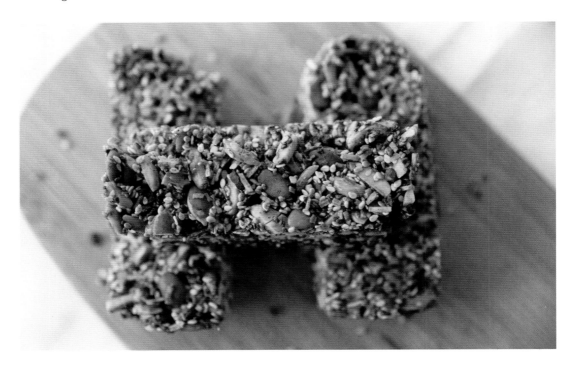

CUCUMBER BOATS

SERVES 1

½ cup (125g) low-fat cottage cheese
1 tsp smoked paprika
1 tsp chopped chives

¼ tsp cayenne pepper
2 slices smoked salmon
2 Lebanese (short) cucumbers

In a bowl, combine the cottage cheese, smoked paprika, chives and cayenne pepper. Season with salt and pepper and give it a good mix.

Wash the cucumbers and remove the ends, then cut them in half lengthways. Spoon the cottage cheese mixture onto each boat and top with smoked salmon.

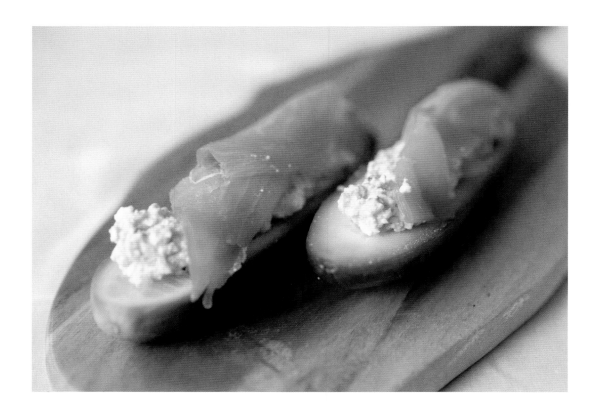

GUACAMOLE CRUNCH

SERVES 2

4 celery stalks

1 small avocado

1 tsp chia seeds

4 thin strips capsicum, chopped into
    small pieces

1 tbsp lemon juice

¼ small red (Spanish) onion, chopped

Remove the ends of the celery stalks and wash celery. In a bowl, mash the avocado with a fork, then add chia seeds, capsicum, lemon juice and onion, and season with salt and pepper. Mix well, then spoon into the hollow of the celery stalks. Crunch and enjoy.

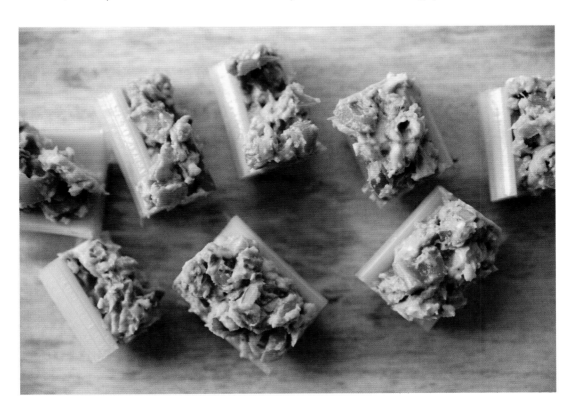

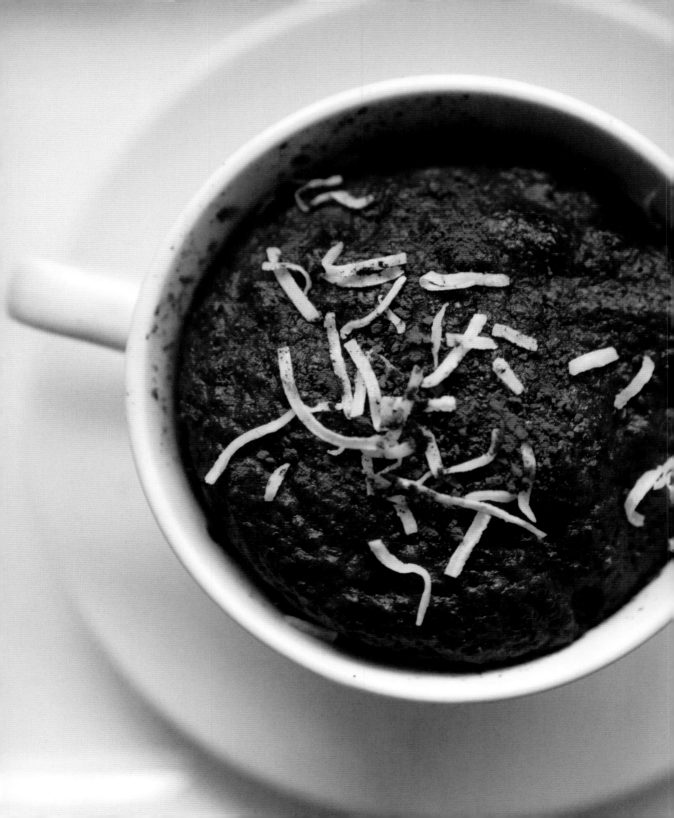

FIVE-MINUTE CHOCOLATE CAKE

If you love chocolate cake, then you'll love this recipe.

SERVES 1

¼ cup (25g) LSA meal (linseed, sunflower seed and almond meal)

1 egg

2 tsp almond butter

2 tsp cacao powder

2 tsp pure maple syrup

1 tsp baking powder

In a small bowl, combine LSA, egg, almond butter, cacao, maple syrup and baking powder. Stir well until all ingredients are combined.

Pour into a microwave-safe coffee mug and microwave for 45–60 seconds on High until cooked. Enjoy!

TURKEY CUPS

SERVES 1

Olive oil spray, for greasing
1 egg
½ tsp smoked paprika
½ tsp curry powder
2 slices turkey breast

Preheat the oven to 180°C. Lightly grease a muffin tin with olive oil spray.

Mix egg, smoked paprika and curry powder together in a small bowl and season with salt and pepper. Line two holes of the muffin tin with slices of turkey and carefully pour the egg mixture on the top. Bake for 10 minutes or until egg is cooked through.

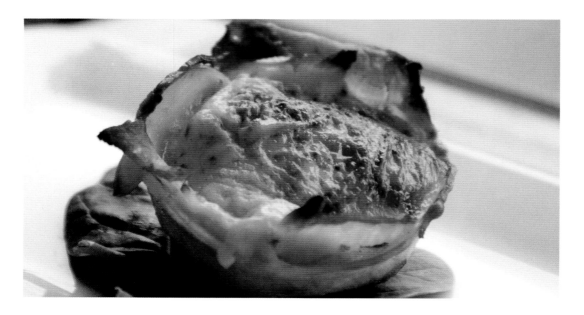

EGG BURRITO

A great combo of protein and good fats that tastes seriously good!

SERVES 1

1 egg
¼ cup (25g) grated parmesan cheese
1 slice turkey breast
1 thin slice avocado

Preheat the sandwich press or use a non-stick frying pan. Whisk the egg and the parmesan together and season with salt and pepper. Pour onto the hot sandwich press and, with the lid up, cook for 3 minutes on each side. Transfer to a plate, top with the slice of turkey and avocado, roll up and enjoy.

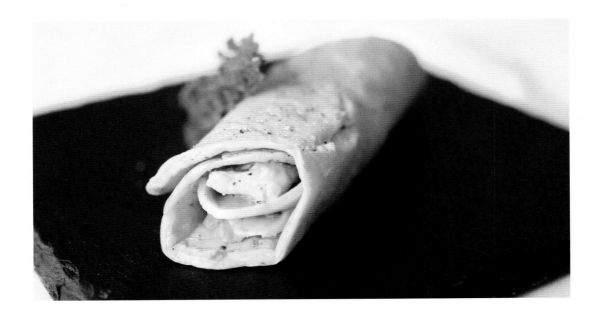

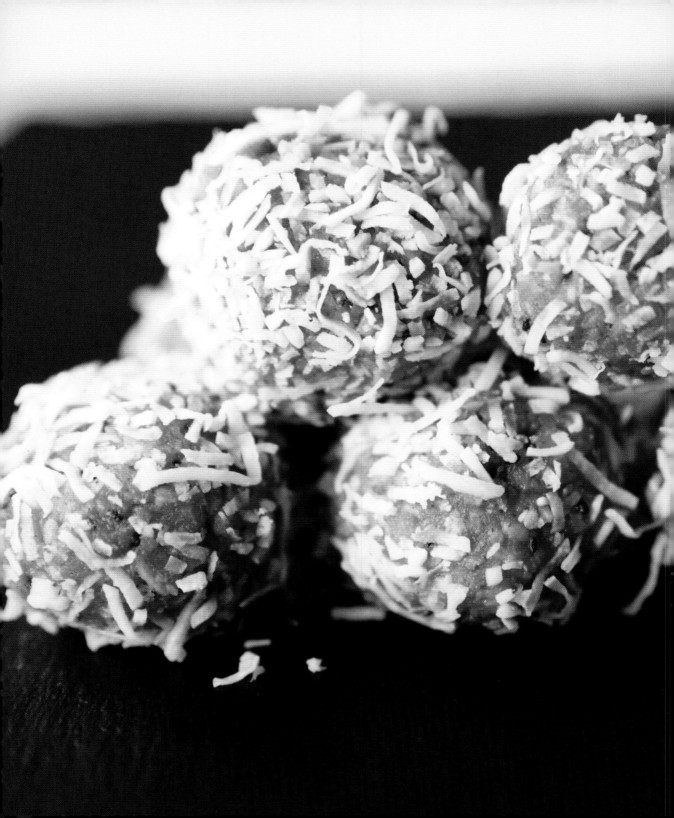

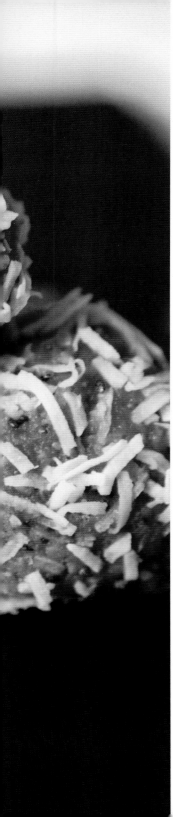

AFTERNOON COFFEE BALLS

MAKES 8–10 BALLS; SERVING SIZE 2 BALLS.

1 cup (100g) almond meal
¼ cup (30g) slivered almonds
2 tsp chia seeds
1 tbsp almond butter
1 tbsp coconut oil
1 shot espresso coffee, cooled
1 tsp vanilla essence
½ cup shredded coconut

Put the almond meal, slivered almonds, chia seeds and almond butter into a food processor.

In a small saucepan, melt coconut oil with the coffee and vanilla over medium heat until combined. Add to the food processor, and blend until all ingredients are well combined.

Put the coconut into a small bowl. Use your hands to form the mixture into balls and then roll each ball in the coconut. Balls should be about the size of a table tennis ball. Place balls on a tray in the fridge to set for at least an hour. Store in an airtight container in the fridge for up to a week.

> **NOTE:** *These are great to have in the fridge for an easy afternoon snack.*

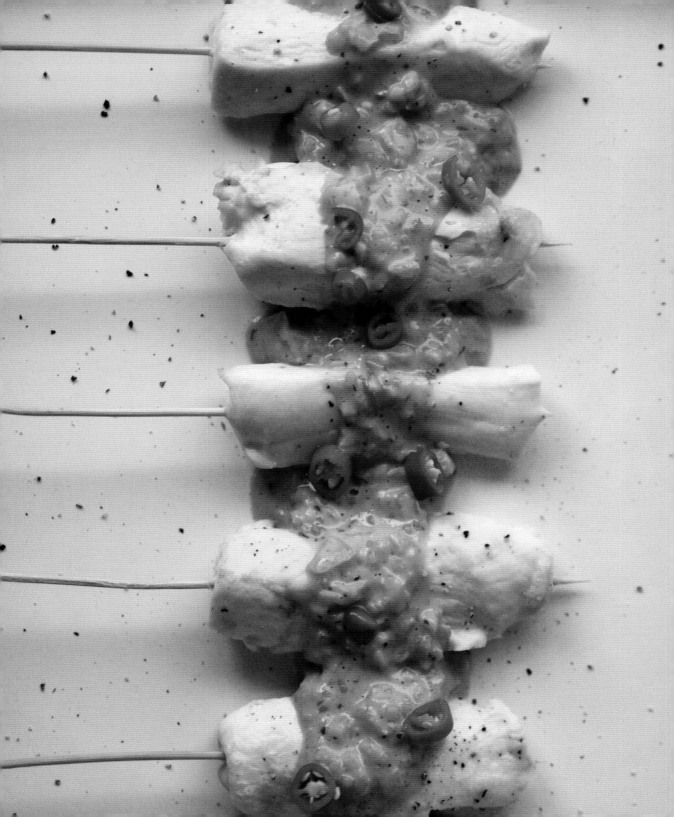

CHICKEN SATAY STICKS

This is a great recipe if you are entertaining. Serve with a nice side salad.

SERVES 2

1 chicken breast

2 tsp olive oil

1 tsp garlic powder

1 onion, finely chopped

1 chilli, finely chopped

1 tsp ground coriander

¼ cup (60g) crunchy peanut butter

1 tsp smoked paprika

1 tbsp lemon juice

1 tbsp tamari (gluten-free soy sauce)

Preheat the oven to 180°C. Soak wooden skewers in water for 15 minutes before using, or use metal skewers. Line a baking dish with baking paper.

Slice chicken into 6cm-long strips. Thread chicken pieces onto skewers and season with salt and pepper. Place in baking dish and cook in the oven for 15 minutes, turning once.

In a frying pan over medium heat, combine the olive oil, garlic, onion, chilli and coriander, and stir-fry until onion is translucent. Add the peanut butter, smoked paprika, lemon juice, tamari and ½ cup water and warm through. Pour the sauce into a blender or food processor and blend until smooth. Pour back into the pan and warm through. Place chicken skewers on a plate, pour the satay sauce over the top and enjoy.

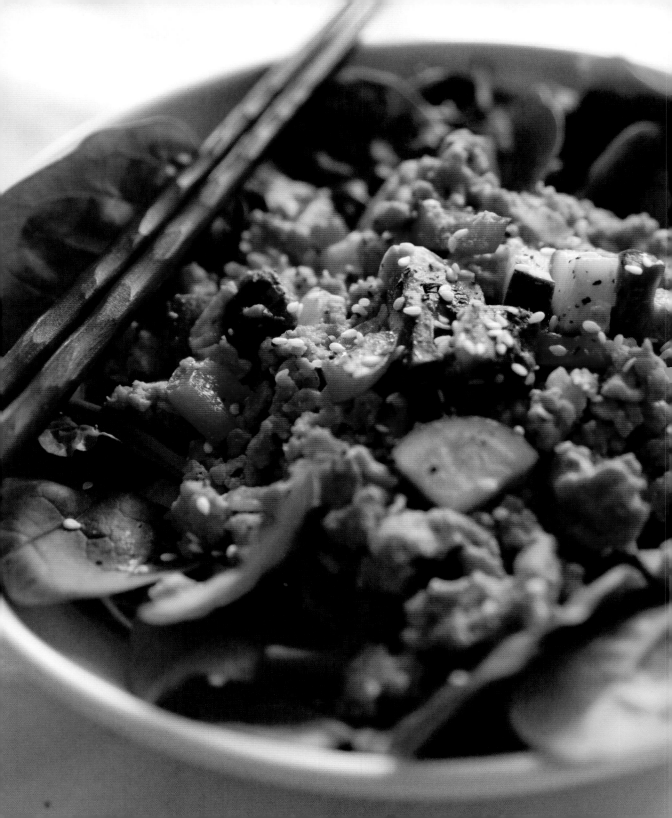

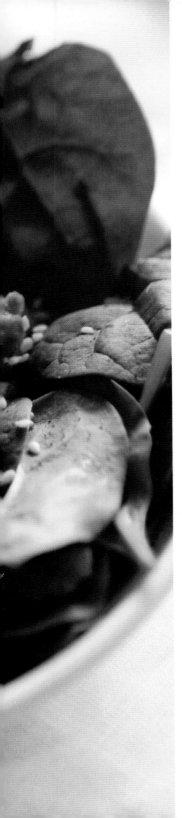

PORK SAN CHOY BAU

SERVES 4

1 tbsp olive oil, plus extra to drizzle
500g pork mince
1 garlic clove, crushed
1 onion, chopped
1 tsp smoked paprika
1 tsp curry powder
1 tsp turmeric
About 2 cups chopped vegies, such as capsicum,
    broccoli, zucchini, mushrooms
1 tbsp oyster sauce
1 egg
Baby spinach and sesame seeds, to serve

Heat olive oil in a frying pan, then add the pork mince, garlic and onion. While the mince is browning, add the smoked paprika, curry powder and turmeric. Stir until mince is cooked.

Add the chopped vegies and oyster sauce and give a good mix. Crack the egg into the pan and mix well, along with a light drizzle of olive oil over the top. Bring to the boil, then reduce heat to low, cover and simmer for 10 minutes before serving.

Put baby spinach in a bowl, top with the mince mixture and sprinkle with sesame seeds. So tasty!

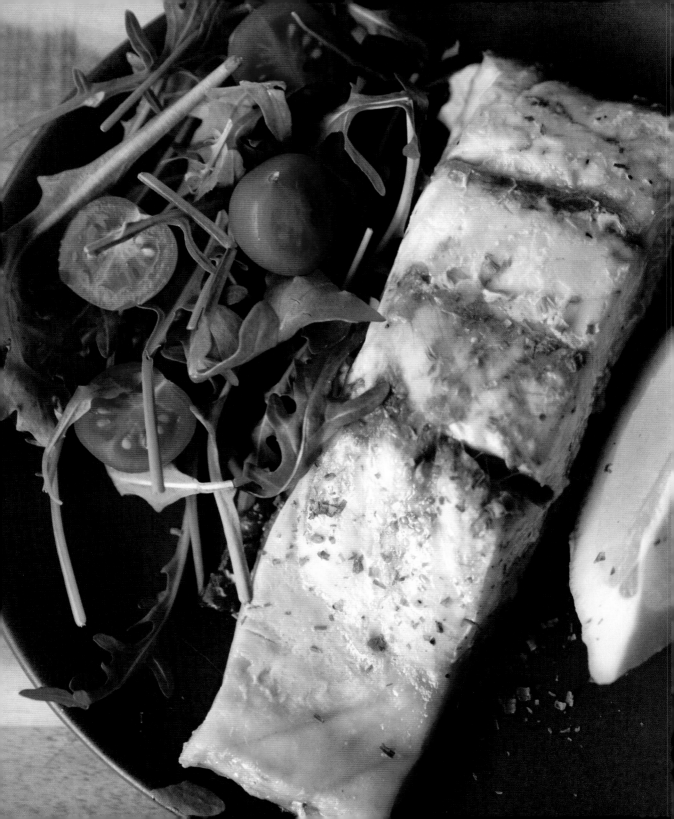

TAMARI AND MAPLE BARRAMUNDI

SERVES 2

¼ cup (60ml) tamari (gluten-free soy sauce)
1 tbsp pure maple syrup
1 tsp lemon juice
2 pieces barramundi fillet or other firm white fresh fish,
    about 100–150g per fillet

Preheat the oven to 180°C.

In a small bowl, mix tamari, maple syrup and lemon juice, season with pepper and stir until combined. Lay out two pieces of foil large enough to completely cover the fish.

Dip barramundi into marinade so it is coated, then place onto foil and wrap up. Place barramundi fillets into baking dish and bake for 20 minutes or until cooked. Serve with vegetables or salad.

> **NOTE:** *You can marinate the fish overnight in the fridge. Tamari is a sweet version of soy sauce and works very well with the maple flavour. Feel free to skip the pre-roasting process and use dry-roasted almonds.*

MINT AND ALMOND ENCRUSTED SALMON

SERVES 2

10 mint leaves
¼ cup (40g) dry-roasted almonds
¼ cup (25g) grated parmesan cheese
1 garlic clove, crushed
2 spring onions, chopped

1 tbsp olive oil
2 pieces of salmon, about
    100–150g per fillet
¼ lemon

Preheat the oven to 180°C. Line a baking tray with foil.

Put the mint, almonds, parmesan, garlic, spring onions and olive oil in a food processor, season with salt and pepper and blend until combined. Lay the salmon on the prepared baking tray and spoon the almond mixture on the top. Bake for 15–20 minutes until opaque. Squeeze lemon over the top. Serve with steamed vegetables.

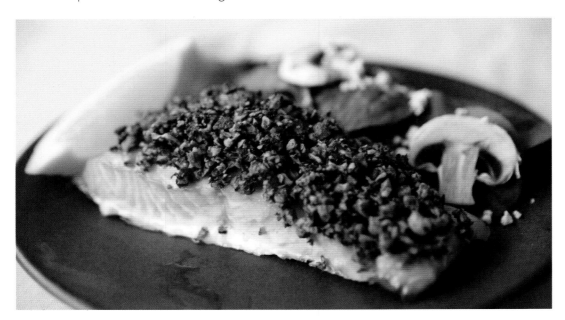

COCONUT CRUMB SCHNITZEL

SERVES 2

½ cup (20g) desiccated coconut
½ cup (55g) LSA (linseed, sunflower seed and almond meal)

¼ cup (25g) grated parmesan cheese
1 egg
4 chicken tenderloins

Preheat the sandwich press or use a non-stick frying pan. In a small bowl combine coconut, LSA and parmesan and mix well.

In a separate bowl, whisk the egg to make an egg wash. Dip chicken into egg wash, then into the coconut mixture and completely coat tenderloins. Place the tenderloins on the sandwich press and cook with the lid down for 5 minutes (cook for 5 minutes each side in a frying pan). Serve with steamed vegetables or salad.

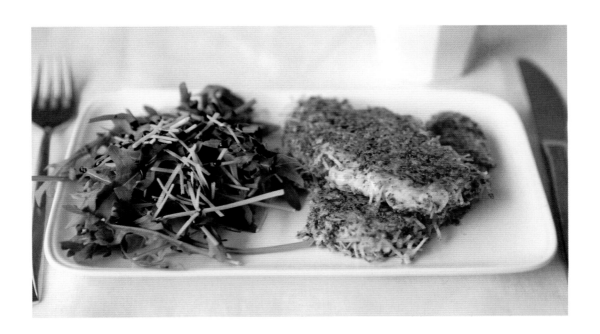

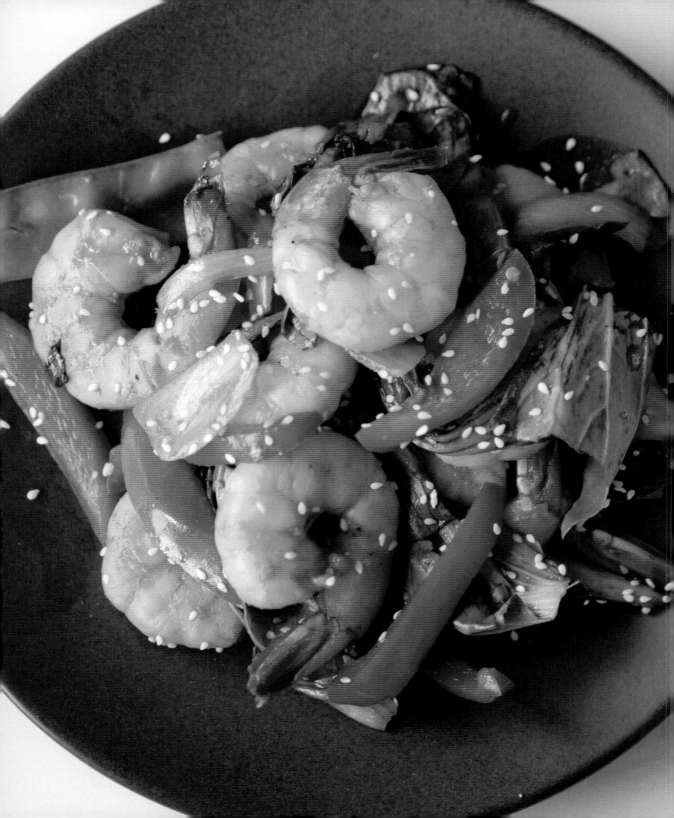

SPICY ASIAN PRAWNS

SERVES 2

½ tsp turmeric

½ tsp cinnamon

1 tsp smoked paprika

¼ cup (60ml) tamari (gluten-free soy sauce)

12 raw prawns, peeled and deveined

Olive oil, for frying

1 onion, chopped

1 garlic clove, crushed

½ tsp ground ginger

1 tsp ground coriander

2 fresh chillies, finely chopped

1 cup snow peas (mangetout)

½ capsicum, sliced into strips

1 head each choy sum (Chinese flowering cabbage) and bok choy (pak choy)

1 tbsp lemon juice

¼ cup (40g) sesame seeds

1 tbsp oyster sauce

In a bowl, combine turmeric, cinnamon, smoked paprika and tamari and mix well. Add the prawns and make sure they are coated. Cover the bowl with plastic wrap and stand in the fridge to marinate for at least 30 minutes.

Heat a splash of olive oil in a frying pan over medium heat, then add the onion, garlic, ginger, coriander and chilli. Stir-fry until onion is translucent. Add the snow peas, capsicum, choy sum, bok choy and oyster sauce and stir-fry for 5 minutes. Add the prawns, season with salt and pepper, then add the lemon juice and sesame seeds. Cook for a further 5 minutes, stirring frequently until prawns are cooked.

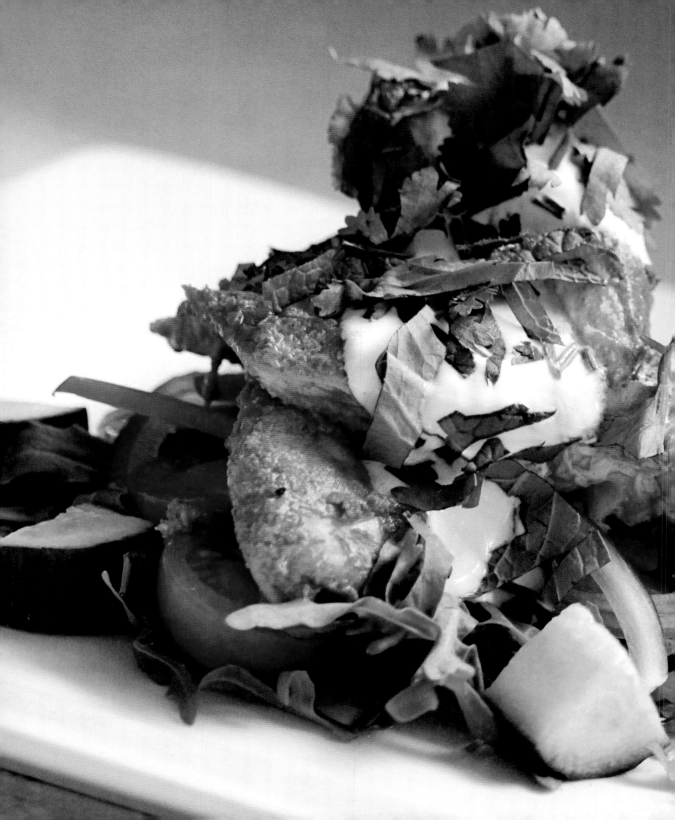

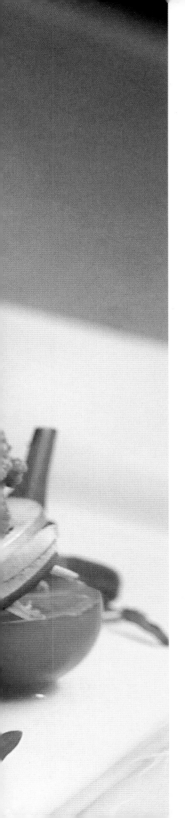

TANDOORI CHICKEN

SERVES 4

3 tbsp tandoori paste
½ cup (125g) Greek-style yoghurt
Juice of ½ lemon
2 large chicken breasts, halved lengthways
1 dollop Greek-style yoghurt, to garnish (optional)
½ cup coriander leaves, to garnish (optional)

SALAD
4 cups (180g) spinach or rocket leaves
1 cup (150g) cherry tomatoes, halved
1 cup (175g) diced cucumber
1 capsicum, deseeded and diced
½ red (Spanish) onion, sliced

Preheat the oven to 180°C. Mix together the tandoori paste, yoghurt and lemon juice in an airtight container, then add the chicken pieces and ensure they are covered with the marinade mixture. Seal with the lid and leave to marinate for 20 minutes.

Line a rectangular baking dish with baking paper, place the chicken pieces in the dish and bake 20–25 minutes until cooked through.

Plate up by arranging the spinach, tomato, cucumber, capsicum and onion on a plate, then placing the chicken on top with a dollop of yoghurt and a scattering of coriander to garnish.

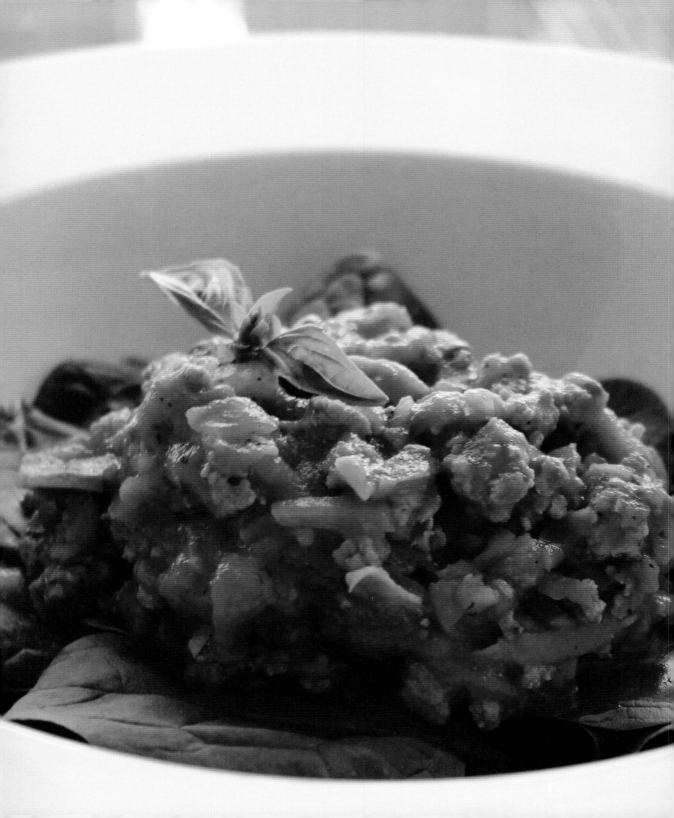

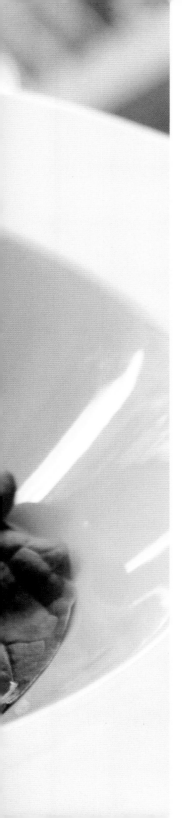

TURKEY BOLOGNESE

SERVES 4

2 tsp olive oil
500g turkey mince
2 garlic cloves, crushed
1 large onion, chopped
1 zucchini (courgette), grated
1 carrot, grated
6 button mushrooms, chopped
400g tin crushed tomatoes
140g tomato paste
1 tsp oregano
Handful of fresh basil leaves
Chilli (optional)

In a heavy-based frying pan with a lid, add the olive oil, turkey mince, garlic and onion, and stir until mince is cooked. Add the zucchini, carrot, mushroom, tomato, tomato paste and oregano, season with salt and pepper and add ½ cup water. Bring to the boil, then tear the basil leaves and add to the pan. Cover and simmer over low heat for about 20 minutes or until vegetables have softened.

Serve on a bed of spinach leaves or over spiralised zucchini noodles.

> **NOTE:** *This is a great staple meal to have up your sleeve during the week: it's quick, easy and delicious.*

MINI RASPBERRY ICE-CREAMS

A portion-controlled treat!

SERVES 14

1 cup (250g) Greek-style yoghurt
½ cup (125g) low-fat cottage cheese
½ cup (70g) frozen raspberries

2 tsp pure maple syrup
1 tsp vanilla essence
14 raspberries, extra, for decoration

Combine the yoghurt, cottage cheese, raspberries, maple syrup and vanilla in a food processor. Blend until smooth, then spoon the mixture into an icetray. Top each ice cube with a raspberry, then place the tray in the freezer for a few hours until mixture sets. Push out a cube and enjoy!

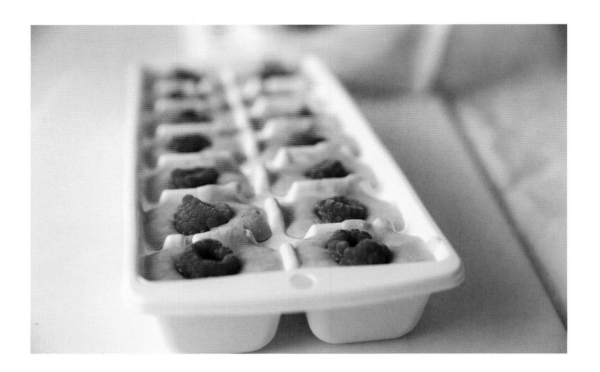

CHOC MINT PROTEIN BALLS

MAKES 10 BALLS

1 cup (100g) LSA meal (linseed, sunflower
   seed and almond meal)
½ cup (50g) rolled oats
10 dates, chopped
1 scoop chocolate protein powder
¼ cup (30g) cacao powder

¼ cup (35g) unsweetened apple sauce
¼ cup (60ml) rice malt syrup
1 tsp peppermint extract
1 tsp vanilla paste
1 tsp chia seeds
½ cup cacao nibs

Place all of the ingredients except the cacao nibs in a food processor, and process until combined.

Put the cacao nibs into a small bowl. Roll mixture into small balls, then roll the balls into the cacao nibs and set out on a tray in the fridge for at least 30 minutes to set.

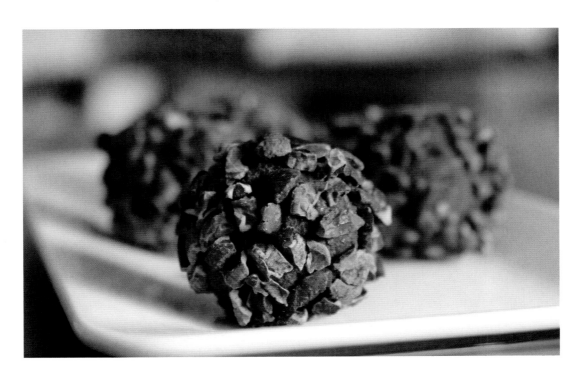

CHOCOLATE GELATO

If you love ice-cream, this is a great treat for you!

SERVES 2

3 bananas
¼ cup (30g) cacao powder
1 tsp vanilla essence
1 cup (140g) frozen mixed berries

Peel the bananas and break them in half; freeze in an airtight container overnight.

Put all of the ingredients into a food processor and blend until smooth and creamy.
Spoon into a bowl and enjoy.

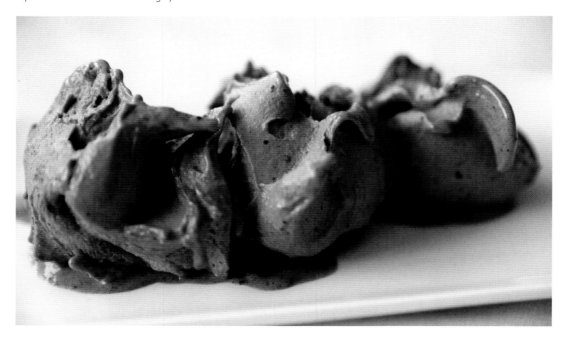

SERIOUSLY GOOD FUDGE

SERVES 9

1 cup (250g) almond butter

½ cup (60g) cacao powder

¼ cup (60ml) pure maple syrup

½ cup (60g) chopped walnuts

Combine the almond butter, cacao powder and maple syrup in a food processor. Transfer to a bowl, add the chopped walnuts and stir to combine.

Line a small square baking tin with baking paper and spoon in the mixture. Using the back of the spoon, spread out the mixture so it is about 2.5 cm thick and a nice square shape. Refrigerate for 2 hours, slice into squares and store in fridge.

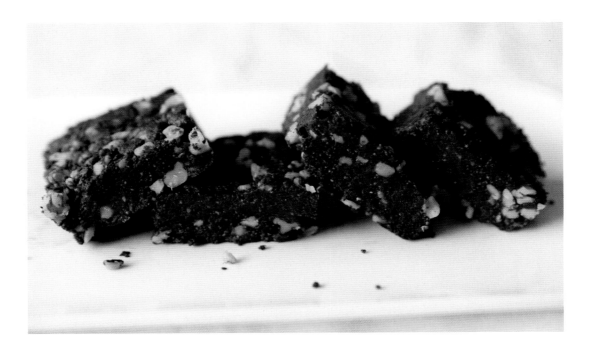

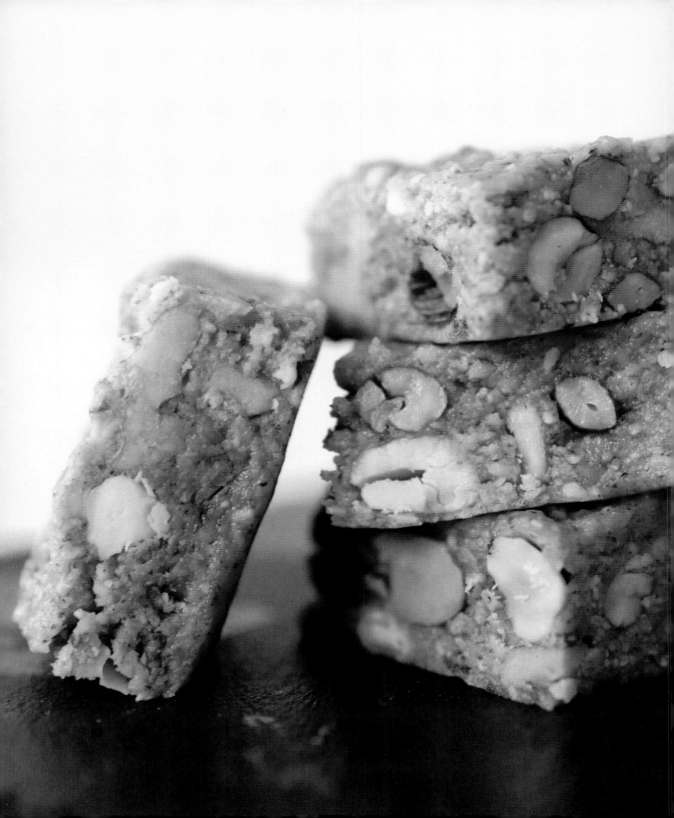

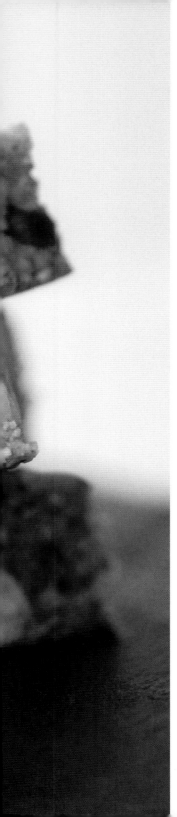

STICKY NUTS

SERVES 4

500g mixed nuts
½ cup (125ml) rice malt syrup
2 tsp pure maple syrup
Pinch of salt

Preheat the oven to 180°C. Line a small square baking tin with baking paper.

Spread 150 g of the nuts (about a third) on a baking tray lined with baking paper and roast in the oven for 10 minutes, but be careful not to burn them!

Put the remaining nuts in a food processor and process until near butter consistency.

In a saucepan over medium heat, put the rice syrup, maple syrup and salt. Stir until syrup takes on a watery consistency. Stir in the nut butter from the food processor and mix well.

Add the roasted nuts to the mixture in the saucepan. Pour into the prepared baking dish and stand in the fridge to set for 30 minutes, then cut into squares.

KIM'S GREEN JUICE

SERVES 1

1 cucumber
4 kale leaves, stems discarded
Handful of spinach leaves
2 celery stalks

1 apple (with skin on)
1 lemon (peeled)
Sliver of ginger (to add a bit of zing)

Wash all the ingredients. Put the cucumber, kale, spinach, celery, apple, lemon and ginger into a juicer. Drink and enjoy!

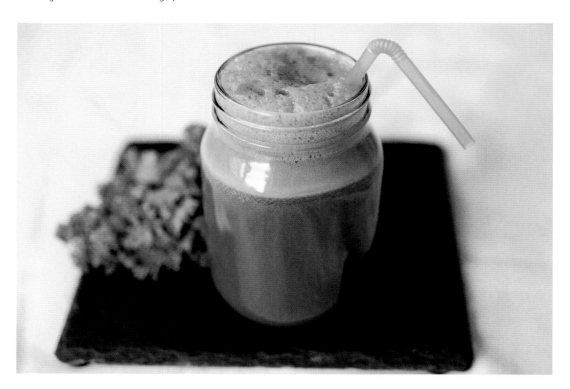

TAMARI ALMONDS

MAKES 1 CUP (15 ALMONDS PER SERVE)

1 cup (155g) almonds
¼ cup (60ml) tamari (gluten-free soy sauce)
2 tbsp pure maple syrup

Pinch of rock salt
Olive oil spray

Preheat the oven to 160°C. Line a baking tray with baking paper, spread almonds evenly on it and pop it into the oven for 7–8 minutes to give them a light roasting.

Combine the tamari, maple syrup and salt in a bowl. Remove the almonds from oven and add to the tamari mixture. Stir to ensure that all almonds are coated. Using a colander, strain the almonds to remove excess tamari mixture.

Spray the baking paper with olive oil spray and spread the coated almonds evenly. Roast for a further 10 minutes (keep an eye on them to ensure they don't burn). Remove almonds and transfer to a clean sheet of baking paper so they don't touch and allow to cool.

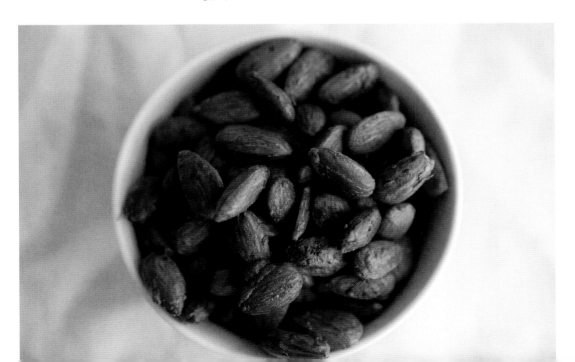

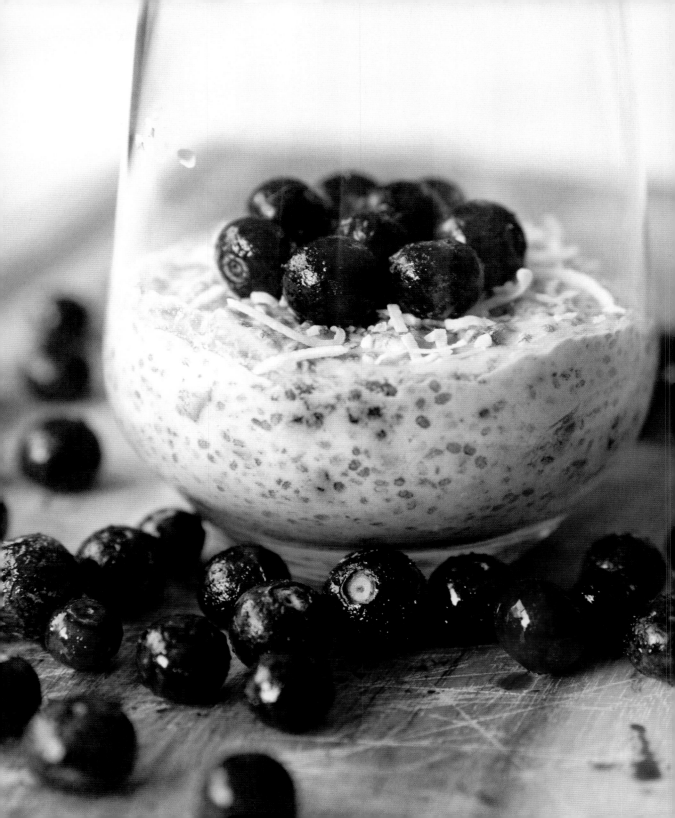

BLUEBERRY CHIA PUDDING

SERVES 2

1 cup (250g) coconut cream
½ cup (80g) blueberries (frozen is fine)
¼ cup (20g) desiccated coconut, plus extra, to garnish
1 tsp vanilla essence
¼ cup chia seeds
¼ cup (40g) blueberries, extra, to garnish

Put the coconut cream, blueberries, coconut and vanilla essence into a food processor and blend until smooth. Transfer to a small bowl, add the chia seeds and mix well.

Pour the mixture into two separate cups or bowls and stir well again. Stand in the fridge to set for a few hours or overnight.

When the puddings have set, top with the extra coconut and blueberries, then sit back and enjoy.

It's never too late to
be a rock star!

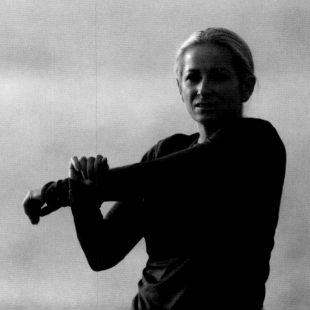

OUR FINAL TEAM TALK

Congratulations! You are now ready to create a fitter, healthier you.

Just before you run out onto the field, I would like to give you a final reminder of the five important principles that will determine your success long term.

These are the tried-and-tested cornerstones of my philosophy that have helped thousands of women achieve their health-and-fitness goals, so write them down and keep them close to you.

Remember the 80:20 rule. Perfection is not required! What IS required is a commitment to being consistent over time.

- **Weight training is your new best friend.**
- **Fuel your body with real food.**
- **Preparation is the key to success.**
- **Surround yourself with positive people who believe in your dreams.**
- **You've got this!**

MY PLANS

It's now time to take action!

The following pages will help you to get organised and create a plan that is achievable for you.

MY GOALS
Write down some short-term goals and then write down some long-term goals, including your BIG scary goal.

MY NUTRITION PLAN
Be really specific and clearly record a list of foods/beverages that you will incorporate into your daily life that are going to fuel your body, as well as a list of foods/beverages that you are now going to try to avoid. Then write down why you are going to make better food choices and why you are going to avoid the foods that hold little to no nutritional value.

MY TRAINING PLAN
Write down how many days you have decided you can train per week, remembering this has to be achievable. List the days you will be training and what training you will be completing on these days. Underneath, write down why training is important to you and what you want to achieve from your training plan.

Once you have written out your three plans, either keep this book in a place where you will see it every day (like your bedside table) or take a copy of the pages and stick them on your fridge or somewhere else you'll see them regularly. These three plans you have created are a fantastic tool to keep you motivated and accountable – use them to your advantage!

MY GOALS

MY NUTRITION PLAN

MY TRAINING PLAN

ACKNOWLEDGMENTS

I vividly remember sitting in our New York hotel room when I first told John that I wanted to write a book. It was early January 2016 and we were on a long-awaited family holiday, finally relaxing after a massive year of work.

It was only a few short weeks later that an email popped into my inbox from Katie at ABC Books, asking me if I would like to collaborate on a book with them. I remember just sitting there and smiling for a good five minutes, as if the universe had just delivered on one of my big crazy goals!

This book wouldn't be possible without the help of some very special people.

Thanks to Katie and the team at ABC Books for believing in me. You guys have been amazing to work with from the start. Writing a book has challenged and stretched me in more ways than I could have imagined but I have loved every minute of it.

To Steve: thank you for helping me create the stunning images for the book, and to Rachel, thanks for the amazing job with hair and make-up.

Alissa: you are a great friend, thanks for turning up on an extremely cold morning at very short notice with no questions asked.

To Mum and Dad: thanks for your total love and support and for looking after Wesley and Chelsea for so many weekends, allowing me the time to write this book.

To Justin and Nic: thanks for the loan of your beautiful new home.

To Christine, Cat and Dean: I will be forever thankful for your grammatical knowledge and your time.

A massive thanks to Ally: I simply don't know what I would do without you!

Most importantly, to John, Wesley and Chelsea: you guys are my world and this project simply would not have happened if it wasn't for your unconditional love, patience and support.

Eat well, lose weight and get healthy with inspiration from Kim Beach, whose down-to-earth approach and achievable advice has already helped thousands of women of all ages.

As a busy mum running a business, Kim Beach understands how difficult it can be to squeeze health and fitness into an over-stuffed schedule, so she's developed solutions that will work for everyone.

Kim's promise is that the long-term answer for a fitter and healthier lifestyle is based around eating well, training hard, staying consistent and, most of all, enjoying the journey. Adopting a practical, real-life approach, *Beach Fit* features:

- Positive nutrition
- Healthy eating for weight loss
- Weekly exercise and eating program
- Step-by-step workouts and plans for weights, HIIT and cardio
- Delicious, healthy recipes that can be prepared in under 20 minutes

Packed with inspiration and expert advice, *Beach Fit* is for anyone who's decided that now is the time to embrace health and fitness in their day-to-day life.

ABC Books   abcbooks.com.au

29.99 / $36.99 CAN
978-0-73-333787-1

52999

9 780733 337871